THE COMPLETE
ILLUSTRATED
GUIDE TO
SHIATSU

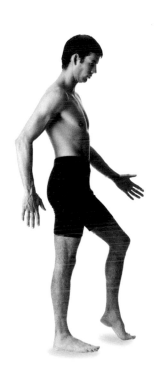

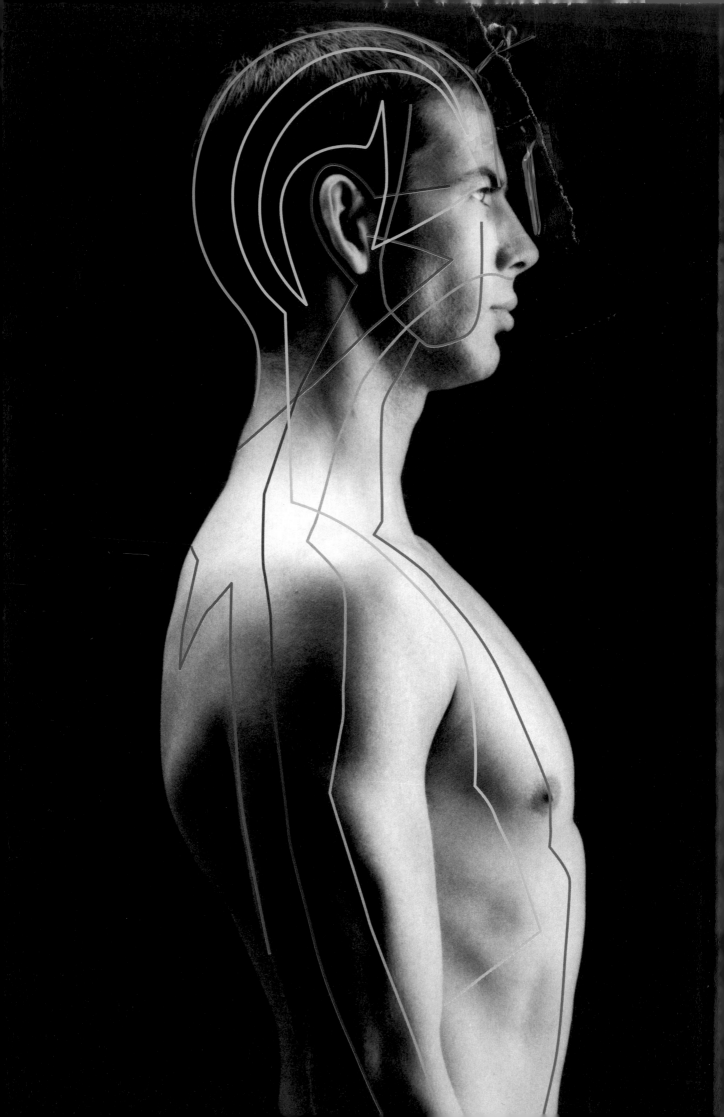

THE COMPLETE
ILLUSTRATED
GUIDE TO
SHIATSU

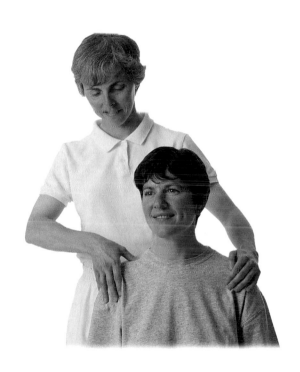

The Japanese Healing Art
of Touch for Health and Fitness

ELAINE LIECHTI

ELEMENT

Shaftesbury, Dorset • Boston, Massachusetts • Melbourne, Victoria

© Element Books 1998
Text © Elaine Liechti 1998

First published in Great Britain 1998 by
ELEMENT BOOKS LIMITED
Shaftesbury, Dorset SP7 8BP

Published in USA in 1998 by
ELEMENT BOOKS INC.
160 North Washington Street
Boston, Massachusetts 02114

Published in Australia in 1998 by
ELEMENT BOOKS LIMITED
and distributed by Penguin Australia Ltd
487 Maroondah Highway, Ringwood, Victoria 3134

NOTE FROM THE PUBLISHER
*Any information given in this book is not intended to
be taken as a replacement for medical advice. Any
person with a condition requiring medical attention
should consult a qualified practitioner or therapist.*

*Designed and created with
The Bridgewater Book Company*

ELEMENT BOOKS LIMITED
Editorial Director: JULIA MCCUTCHEN
Senior Commissioning Editor: CARO NESS
Production Director: ROGER LANE
Senior Production Controller: SARAH GOLDEN

THE BRIDGEWATER BOOK COMPANY
Art Director: PETER BRIDGEWATER
Designers: GLYN BRIDGEWATER, JANE LANAWAY
Managing Editor: ANNE TOWNLEY
Editor: NICKY ADAMSON
Page make-up: CHRIS LANAWAY
Picture research: VANESSA FLETCHER
Three-dimensional models: MARK JAMIESON
Studio photography: GUY RYECART, IAN PARSONS
Illustrators: MICHAEL COURTENAY, IVAN HISSEY,
ANDREW KULMAN

Repro by Appletone Graphics, Bournemouth
Printed and bound by Butler and Tanner, Frome

British Library Cataloguing in
Publication data available

Library of Congress Cataloguing in
Publication data available

Acknowledgements

The publishers wish to thank the following for the use of
pictures:
Bridgeman Art Library: 22TL, 22TL, 86R
Fortean Picture Library: 89BL
Hutchison: 29T, 29B
Image Bank: 63CL
Images Colour Library: 18
Oxford Scientific Films: 152T
Science Photo Library: 52R
Wellcome Institute Library: 12–13T
Zefa Picture Library: 48, 49BR, 51L, 51R, 57col.4, 85TR, 86L
89B, 158L, 159CR, 159C, 186T, 186B

Special thanks go to
Lily Adams, Mays Al-Ali, Maria Anderson, Philip Auchinvole,
Simon Balley, Janine Bennett, Jonathan Henry Brook, Stephanie
Brotherstone, Adam Carne, Alan Carne, Rob Chappell, Stephen
Danes, Rebecca Drury, Carly Evans, Christina Fagarazzi, Cathy
Glendinning, Wendy Grantley-Oxberry, Paul Harley, Deborah
Heath, Dee James, Bert Johnson, Mette Lauritzen, Kay
Macmullan, Jack Martin, Denise McCullough, Jim Mclean,
Norma McLean, Lisa Montague, Mark Nailer, Elin Osmond,
Clare Packman, Anna Rawson, Caron Riley, Sheila Sword,
Helen Tookey, Derek Watts, Louise Webster, Louise Williams
for help with photography

Solutions, Hove, Bright Ideas, Lewes, Blackbrooks Garden
Centre, Sedlescombe, Pine Secrets, Brighton, Gunn and Bone
Futons, Innerliethen, Scotland
for help with properties

The acupoint stimulator is available from Acumedic Ltd,
101–103 Camden High Street, London NW1 7JN

Author's Acknowledgements

I would like to acknowledge my teachers, my clients, and
especially my students, who are a constant source of inspiration.
I am grateful to my colleagues in the Glasgow School of Shiatsu,
especially Hilary Crook, whose friendship and efficiency are
invaluable to me. My heartfelt thanks go to my parents, Geoff
and Athalie Carter, for their encouragement and for baby-sitting
my young son, Christopher, often at short notice. Most of all I
would like to thank my husband, John, and my daughter, Cora,
for their love, support, and understanding.

ISBN 1 86204 178 4

Contents

PART 1
WHAT IS SHIATSU?

PART 2
THE HISTORY OF SHIATSU

PART 3
SHIATSU TODAY

PART 4
HOW SHIATSU WORKS

PART 5
THE TECHNIQUES OF SHIATSU

PART 6
THE SHIATSU SEQUENCE

PART 7
RELATED EXERCISES
AND SELF-HELP MEASURES

PART 8
TAKING IT FURTHER

How to use this Book

The Complete Illustrated Guide to Shiatsu provides a detailed introduction to this healing art, which uses the power of touch and pressure to provide physical and emotional healing. The book gives an account of the history and development of Shiatsu, from its origins in Japan to the growth of modern methods, especially Zen Shiatsu which forms the basis for the techniques given here.

After giving essential background information on the concept of Ki energy, and how its flow through the body can be directed to help with healing, the book discusses Five Element Theory, Yin Yang and the idea of Kyo and Jitsu, as well as the importance of the meridians as the pathways of Ki. It also introduces the Tsubo – key points on the meridians that have a particular function in controlling the flow of Ki to different body parts and organs.

The background theory is put into practice in the Basic Sequence, which uses step-by-step instructions to guide the reader through a complete program of Shiatsu treatment for the whole body. Further chapters provide techniques for Do-In (self-Shiatsu), treatments for specific conditions, and advice on how to approach further instruction toward full practitioner status.

STANDARD MERIDIAN ABBREVIATIONS

The Shiatsu meridians each have specific names: Bladder, Gall Bladder, Small Intestine, and so on. These names are given in full in the text, but in referring to the tsubo points that are worked to alleviate specific conditions the standard Shiatsu abbreviations have been used. These take the form of two letters and a number that identify the location of each point. A full listing of these locations is given on page 186. The standard abbreviations are ST: Stomach; BL: Bladder; LU: Lung; LI: Large Intestine; SI: Small Intestine; KD: Kidney; BL: BLadder; LIV: Liver; GB: Gall Bladder; SP: Spleen; HT: Heart; TH: Triple Heater; HG: Heart Governor.

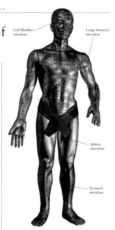

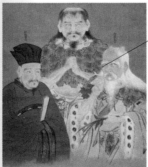

introduction to the influence of oriental philosophy

running text traces the roots of meridian theory

illustrations are carefully chosen to show the historical background

LEFT *The first part of the book places Shiatsu in its proper historical context.*

accurately drawn meridian maps show how Ki energy runs through the body

color coding differentiates separate meridians

RIGHT *The importance of the meridian system to Shiatsu is reflected in the detailed body maps provided throughout the book which show the complex Ki pathways.*

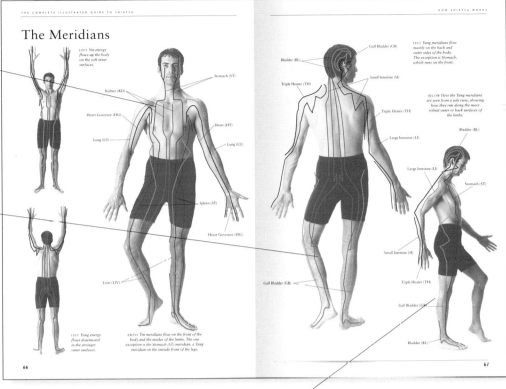

individual meridians to be activated are highlighted throughout the Basic Sequence

each exercise is illustrated, with annotation to pinpoint particular Tsubo, meridians, and muscles

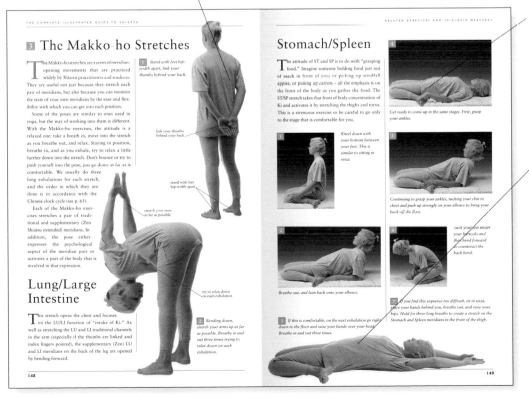

clear photographs take the reader through each step of the sequence

advanced techniques are also illustrated so that all levels of ability can be accommodated

LEFT *The Basic Sequence section is the heart of the book where the techniques of Shiatsu are demonstrated through clear text and photographs.*

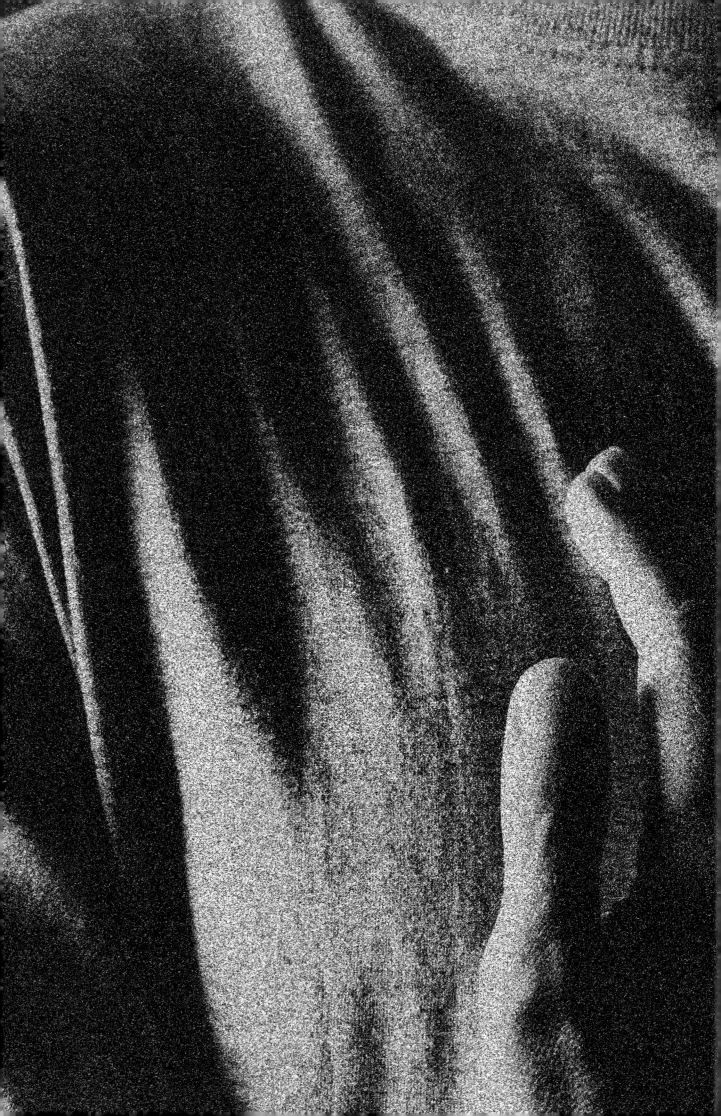

WHAT IS SHIATSU?

The healing art of Shiatsu uses physical pressure and meridian stretches to work on the body's energetic systems to promote health and spiritual well-being.

Shiatsu as Therapy

Shiatsu is a healing art originating in Japan that uses the power of touch and pressure to enable each of us to contact our own abilities for self-healing. In a Shiatsu session the practitioner uses pressure with his or her thumbs, fingers, palms, and sometimes elbows, knees, and feet, to induce deep relaxation and a feeling of well-being. It is sometimes a dynamic, sometimes a more static form of therapy, involving pressure on and stretching of the limbs and torso, kneading and releasing tight muscles, and supporting areas of weakness. To receive Shiatsu is deeply relaxing and yet invigorating, leaving the receiver with a feeling of tranquillity and a sense of being in touch with every part of one's body. Giving Shiatsu is like performing a moving meditation and leaves the practitioner feeling as balanced and energized as the receiver.

Shiatsu was developed from traditional oriental massage and, in common with acupuncture and other oriental therapies, it works upon the body's energetic system using the network of meridians or energy pathways that relate to the functioning of the internal organs as well as our emotional, psychological, and spiritual harmony. The concept of the body as an "energetic" organism comes from ancient Chinese thought, and through centuries of experience and study, has evolved into a system of medical

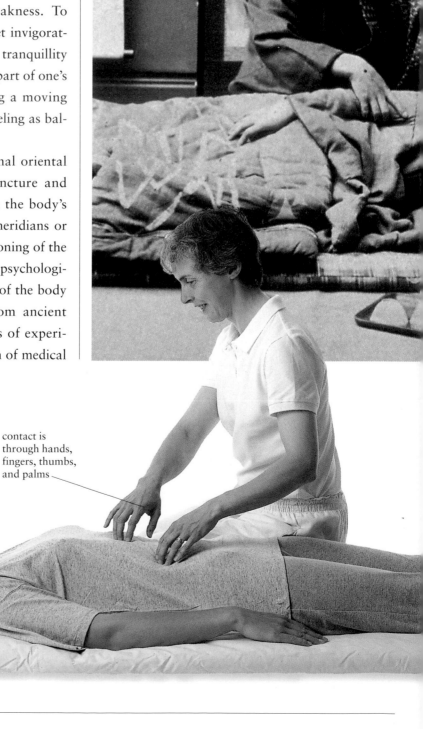

RIGHT *Modern Shiatsu creates a unique bond between practitioner and receiver.*

contact is through hands, fingers, thumbs, and palms

receiver benefits both physically and mentally

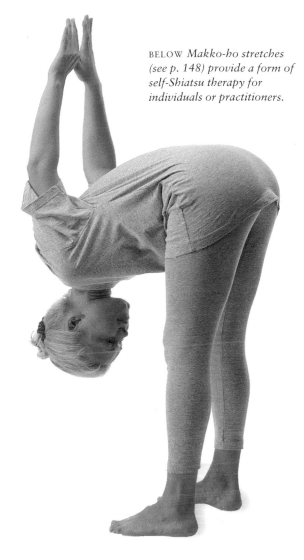

BELOW *Makko-ho stretches (see p. 148) provide a form of self-Shiatsu therapy for individuals or practitioners.*

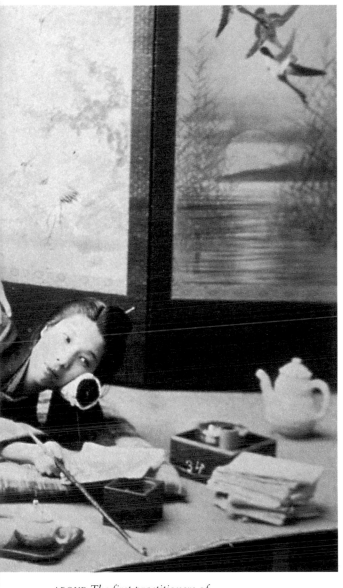

ABOVE *The first practitioners of Shiatsu in Japan were blind since it was thought their sense of touch was heightened.*

soft clothing promotes relaxation and prevents inhibiting shyness

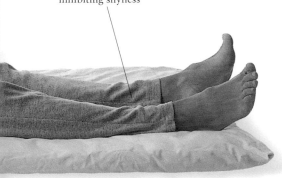

theory that is both rich and poetic. Energy, known as Ki in Japanese (Qi in Chinese), flows throughout the body like a system of rivers and canals. Things may happen to upset the smooth flow of Ki, causing blockages or dams in some areas, and weaknesses or stagnant pools in others. These blockages or weaknesses in turn may lead to physical symptoms, to psychological or emotional disturbances, or simply to a feeling that "things are just not quite right."

Shiatsu uses physical pressure and meridian stretches to unblock the dams – which show up as tight muscles and areas of stiffness – and revitalize the empty areas – which may feel cold, weak, or just needing to be held. Oriental medical theory provides a framework by which the practitioner can assess the body's energetic state and needs, and can explain why the body holds tension in certain areas or points and feels weak in others.

The Power of Touch

The techniques used in Shiatsu are both simple and profound. We are all familiar with "the healing power of touch." Every mother knows that a kiss and "let Mommy rub it better" is more effective than a Bandaid; athletes find that immediate local massage can do much to restore a pulled muscle, and who has not felt better for a hug in times of emotional stress? Yet although we are aware at a common sense level that we need touch, our society has largely educated that intuitive feeling out of us, so that it is not socially acceptable to ask for or give physical contact unless in an extreme or traumatic situation.

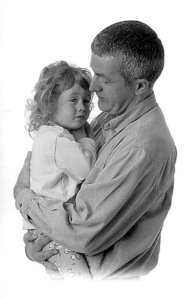

ABOVE *Physical contact is important for well-being; it's an automatic response to want to cuddle an unhappy child.*

All forms of bodywork and massage can fulfill the need for touch, but Shiatsu is particularly applicable and practical in an everyday setting for a variety of reasons. One important aspect is that the receiver remains clothed during the treatment. In a society where we have inhibitions about being touched, removing clothes is a further challenge that makes the receiver feel uncomfortably vulnerable. Secondly, the slow and sustained holding pressure that characterizes Shiatsu actively encourages conscious relaxation. This allows the physiological mechanisms governing muscle tension to release more efficiently than with some other forms of bodywork. Thirdly, Shiatsu is very practical: it requires no special equipment, just a blanket or mat on the floor, and peace and quiet. And fourthly, although Shiatsu can be used

to treat a number of serious complaints when practiced by a fully trained therapist, the basics can be mastered by anyone taking introductory classes. The knowledge gained at this level is sufficient to ease everyday aches, pains, and minor problems in a family or work setting or between friends. Indeed, this is possibly one of the greatest strengths of Shiatsu. In Japan, Shiatsu is widely used as a home remedy, and there is no reason why, as Shiatsu receives wider international recognition, this should not be the case in Western society. In this context it can do a great deal to strengthen human relationships, relieve the stress of modern living, and provide compassionate support in times of trouble.

BELOW *Shiatsu is a particularly comfortable form of physical contact as it is slow and sustained.*

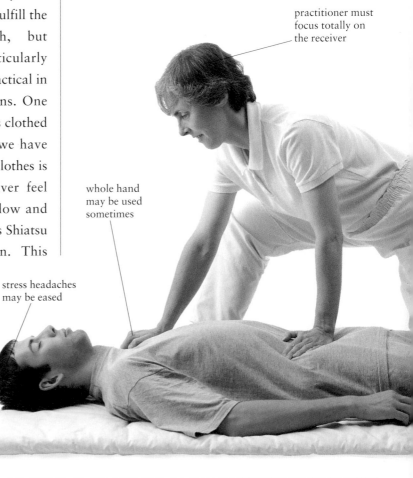

practitioner must focus totally on the receiver

whole hand may be used sometimes

stress headaches may be eased

Prevention and Treatment

Like other natural healing and alternative therapies, Shiatsu is concerned with preventative measures. Shiatsu keeps the body healthy, flexible, and in balance, as well as monitoring the energetic changes that may be precursors of sickness. In the oriental view, an imbalance of Ki develops before the symptoms of illness occur. Regular Shiatsu treatment can help to pinpoint any patterns of imbalance in the body's Ki structure by ironing out those disturbances before they become entrenched. In the case of people already suffering from health problems, Shiatsu can be of great benefit, both as a discipline in its own right and in concert with other complementary and orthodox treatments.

An experienced Shiatsu practitioner may explain the imbalance in terms of oriental theory to help the patient understand his or her condition. Some practitioners suggest dietary and lifestyle changes to aid healing. Stretching exercises and points to press may form part of a patient's "homework" to sustain the effect of the treatment between sessions.

Many people find that a Shiatsu session once a month, or at the change of the seasons, is a useful part of their general health maintenance programme, rather like having a medical or dental check-up. So often people comment, "I didn't know that part was sore until you pressed it," or they find that unexpressed emotions can be discharged in the "safe space" of the treatment room. The physical and psychological release obtained during Shiatsu can make life more comfortable and in some cases can make it bearable.

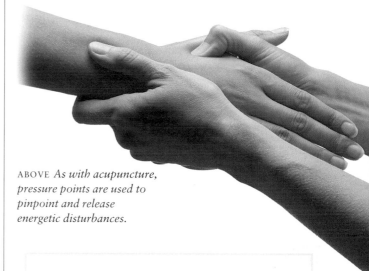

ABOVE *As with acupuncture, pressure points are used to pinpoint and release energetic disturbances.*

SHIATSU CAN HELP

Many conditions are particularly suitable for Shiatsu treatment, including headaches and migraine, acute and chronic back pain (especially if of muscular origin), sciatica, muscular stiffness and injuries, some forms of arthritis, and rheumatic complaints. Working as it does on the body's internal organs, Shiatsu can also have a role in the treatment of digestive and intestinal disorders and circulatory, respiratory, and reproductive problems. Because Shiatsu works on relaxing the body at a deep level and contacting the more subtle aspects of one's energetic makeup, it can also help in the treatment of anxiety, tension, depression, and emotional instability.

ABOVE *Shiatsu can relieve the stiffness of old age.*

RIGHT *Shiatsu benefits professionals who experience physical stress, such as dancers or athletes.*

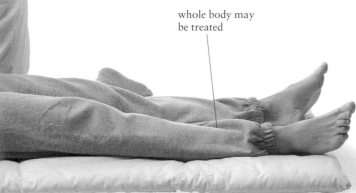

whole body may be treated

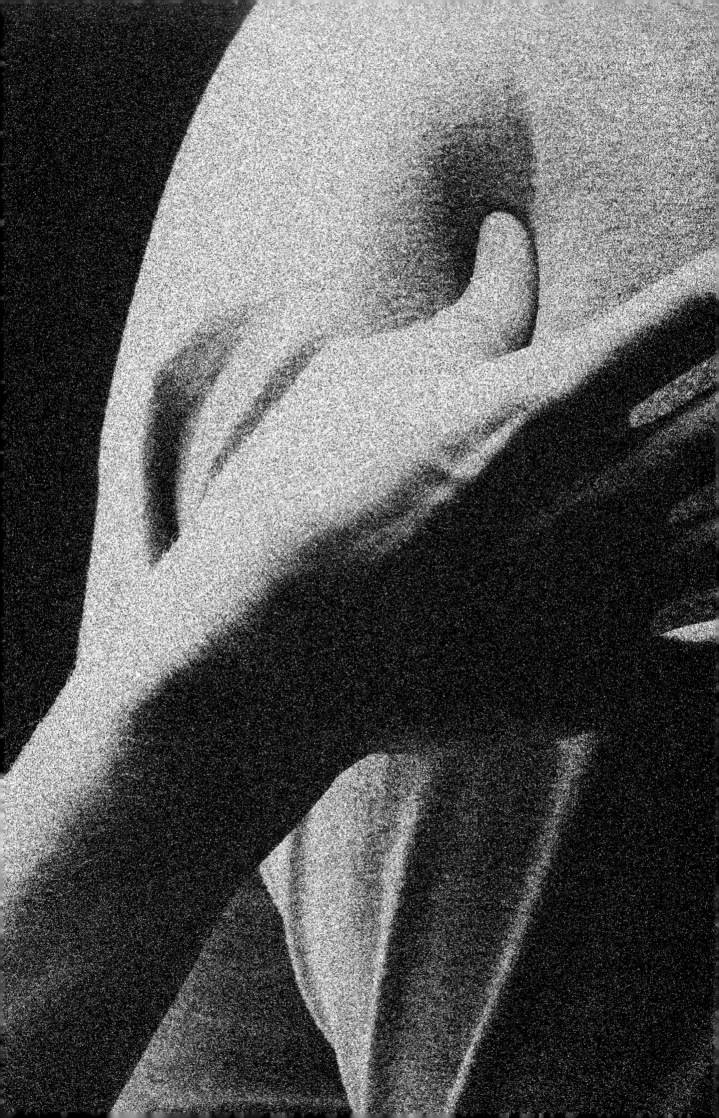

THE HISTORY OF SHIATSU

Shiatsu's history is closely bound to its origins in ancient oriental principles of medicine, and their close association with philosophy, culture, and spirituality.

⊞ The Influence of Chinese Medicine

To discover the historical roots of Shiatsu we must go back to ancient China, where the basic principles of all forms of oriental medicine originated. It must first of all be clearly understood that oriental medical theory arose from, and is part of, Chinese philosophy. In the West we tend to think of medicine as being a distinct discipline, having nothing in common with, for example, politics, philosophy, or art. In contrast, the theories underpinning oriental medicine are the same as those underpinning Chinese thought, culture, art, religion, philosophy, politics, and so on. In other words, the ancient Chinese formulated certain principles that were perceived as universal truths and they applied those principles to the realm of medicine. It is probably this very fact that has ensured the continuation of the practice of oriental medicine in largely the same form for centuries, although it must be said that modern Chinese teaching tends to ignore some of the more esoteric and philosophical aspects.

THE EARLY HISTORY OF ORIENTAL MEDICINE

The very early history of oriental medicine is so old as to be clouded in uncertainty and a degree of myth, but the practice of acupuncture is known to date from before 2500 B.C.E. A bronze model showing acupuncture points and meridians has been dated at around 860 C.E. The oldest existing medical text is the Huang Ti Nei Ching Su Wen (usually abbreviated to Nei Ching) – *The Yellow Emperor's Classic of Internal Medicine*, said to have been written by Huang Ti, the legendary Yellow Emperor who died about 2598 B.C.E. This work is still a respected and oft-quoted source and is an important area of study in modern acupuncture teaching. There is scholarly debate, however, as to the exact authorship and dating of the work. The earliest mention of the Nei Ching is made during the first part of the Han Dynasty (206 B.C.E.–25 C.E.). Later editions and

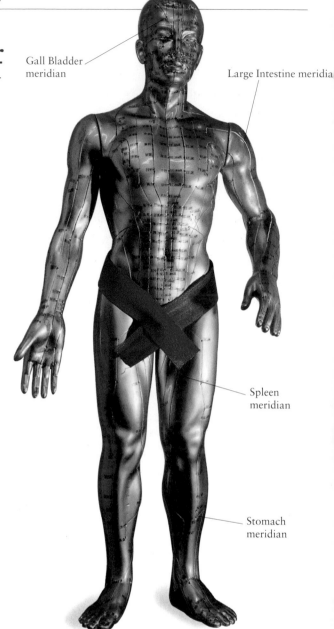

Gall Bladder meridian

Large Intestine meridian

Spleen meridian

Stomach meridian

ABOVE *Chinese bronze model of the "Acupuncture Man" (Zeng Jui Toing Ren), with the main energy line and healing points picked out in relief.*

commentaries further cloud the original date and authorship, however, as Ilza Veith states in the introduction to the University of California Press edition of the Nei Ching: it is fair to assume that a great part of the text existed during the Han Dynasty, and that much of it is of considerably older origin, possibly handed down by oral tradition from China's earliest history thousands of years ago.

The text is in the form of a dialogue between the Yellow Emperor and his minister Ch'i Po, in which the Emperor asks questions on the subject of health and medicine, and Ch'i Po replies at length, drawing upon medical theory and philosophical beliefs.

This form of writing makes it possible to enlarge the scope of the work far beyond that of a medical textbook and to change it into a treatise on general ethics and regimen of life, and to include in it the prevailing Chinese religious beliefs. This combination is, as a matter of fact, the only way in which early Chinese medical thinking could be expressed, for medicine was but a part of philosophy and religion, both of which propounded oneness with nature, i.e., the universe.

The Nei Ching makes reference to the geographical factors that affected the early development of medical techniques in China. There were two distinct branches of medicine. The Northern method, from the Yellow River basin where vegetation was sparse and the climate cold, was comprised predominantly of acupuncture, moxibustion, and massage. The Southern tradition originated in the Yangtze River region, where the climate was warmer and there was a variety of abundant plant life, enabling the people in this area to use the roots, leaves, and bark of plants and other substances to form a very comprehensive system of herbal treatment. Both traditions arose from the climatic and environmental influences of their respective regions and in response to the kinds of illnesses that were common in those areas.

The Nei Ching goes into detail about which diseases are found in which area and what the appropriate form of treatment is. It mentions the people of the East, whose diet of fish and salt causes them to "burn within" producing ulcers, which are best treated with flint needle acupuncture. The people of the North are subject to many diseases because of the cold, and moxibustion is the appropriate remedy. Moxibustion is the burning of mugwort over particular points and areas in order to introduce heat and stimulate local circulation. Each area, North, South, East, West, and Center, is noted. Massage is the specific treatment for the people of the Central region of China.

"The region of the center, the Earth, is level and moist. Everything that is created by the Universe meets in the center and is absorbed by the Earth.

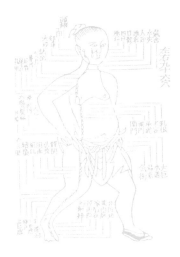

ABOVE *An eighteenth-century drawing of the "sunlight" vessel of the stomach, as described in* The Yellow Emperor's Classic of Internal Medicine, *showing 48 acupuncture spots.*

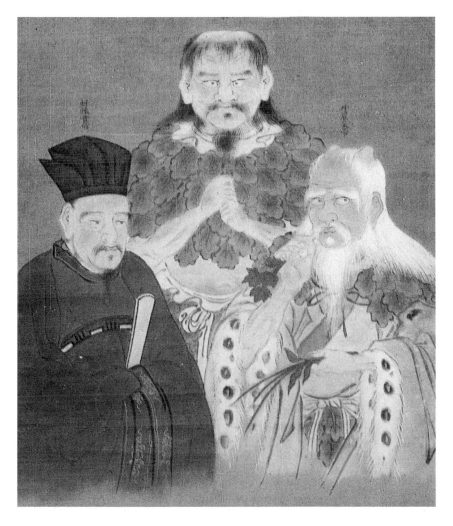

LEFT *The three legendary Emperors, Fu Hsi, Shen Nung, and Huang Ti, who are supposed to have founded the art of healing nearly 5,000 years ago.*

The people of the regions of the center eat mixed food and do not (suffer or weary at their) toil. Their diseases are many: they suffer from complete paralysis and chills and fever. These diseases are most fittingly treated with breathing exercises, massage of the skin and flesh, and exercises of the hands and feet. Hence the treatment with breathing exercises, massage and exercises of the limbs has its origin in the center regions."

FROM *THE YELLOW EMPEROR'S CLASSIC OF INTERNAL MEDICINE.*

The Northern and Southern methods were brought together to form a comprehensive theory of medicine under the Han Dynasty (206 B.C.E.–220 C.E.) when China was unified.

Massage was thus from the very first acknowledged as one of the four classical forms of medical treatment, along with acupuncture, moxibustion, and herbalism. The form of massage used was called Anmo or Mo (or Anma in Japan) and employed a combination of rubbing and pressing stiff and sore areas. (Modern Chinese massage is known as Tui Na.) The discovery of which areas and points were effective for which conditions no doubt evolved over centuries of experience, observation, and trial and error. This knowledge would have been largely transmitted by word of mouth from doctor to apprentice, mother to daughter, and so on. Evidence of this lies in the fact that acupuncture has been well documented from the earliest writings, but textbooks on Anmo methods are relatively rare, and often incorporate breathing and movement exercises such as Qi Gong, Tai Chi, and Tao Yin. In *The History of Scientific Thought*, volume 2, Joseph Needham writes that Chinese massage (Mo) generated a large body of works, the principal ones being *The Manual of Nourishing the Life by Gymnastics* (date unknown) and *Eight Chapters on Putting Oneself in Accord with the Life Force* by Kao Lien, dated 1591.

ABOVE *Needles used for Chinese acupuncture (actual size).*

BELOW *Moxibustion – the technique of warming an affected area by burning the herb mugwort over it – was described in the Nei Ching, the Yellow Emperor's book.*

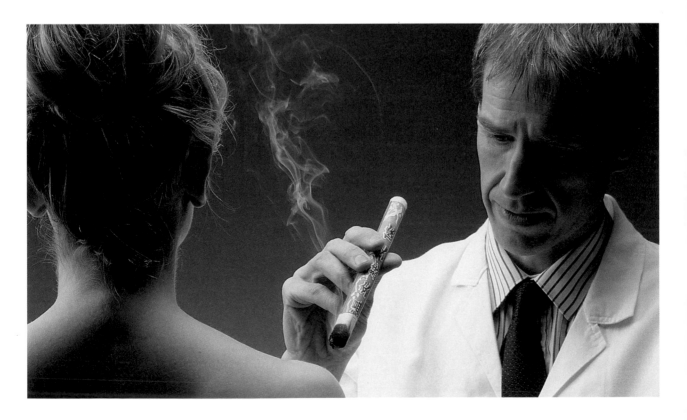

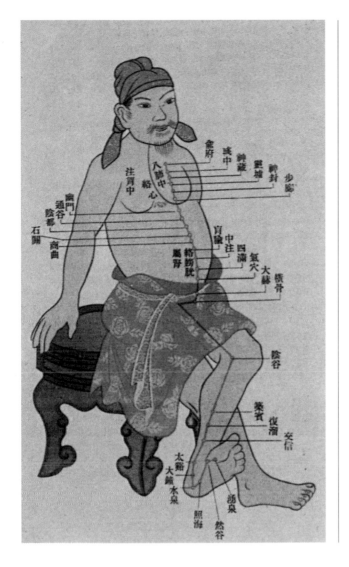

There are those who believe that massage using the body's energetic flows actually predates acupuncture. Certainly from a practical point of view it seems to make sense that a system of pressing and rubbing the body with the hands should develop before the use of tools (that is, acupuncture needles). It is also interesting that modern-day acupuncturists are usually taught manual palpation of points and massage in order to familiarize them with the body's energy before they are allowed to use needles. Possible evidence for the theory that acupuncture developed later than massage and moxibustion comes in the relatively recent discovery of a text dated before the Nei Ching, in which "No points are mentioned, just entire Meridians, portraying zones of influence needing stimulation by moxibustion.

This evidence suggests Meridians existed before points." (T. Kaptchuk, *Chinese Medicine: The Web That Has No Weaver*.) What is meant here is that knowledge of meridians and the application of technique to the meridians existed before knowledge of the use of points.

LEFT *Chinese painting of the Kidney vessel, showing the acupuncture points.*

THE YELLOW EMPEROR

Huang Ti, the Yellow Emperor, is a figure of great importance in China's mythology and history. Mystery and legend cloud the exact details of his reign and achievements; indeed there is even doubt in some modern circles as to his actual existence. However, it is generally accepted that he was the third of China's first five legendary emperors and that he lived for 100 years, ruling between 2696 and 2598 B.C.E., just after the completion of the Great Pyramids in Egypt.

The first book of the Mei Ching Su Wu, *The Yellow Emperor's Classic of Internal Medicine*, begins: "In ancient times when the Yellow Emperor was born he was endowed with divine talents; while yet in early infancy he could speak; while still very young he was quick of apprehension and penetrating; when he was grown up he was sincere and comprehending; when he became perfect he ascended into heaven." (This quotation is taken from the translation by Elza Veith, University of California Press.)

In addition to his medical expertise, Huang Ti is attributed with the invention of wheeled carts and carriages, the development of the Chinese 60 year cycle calendar, and the design of pottery and musical instruments. Legend says that his wife discovered how to rear silkworms and this began the Chinese silk industry. At the end of the Yellow Emperor's life a phoenix and a unicorn are said to have appeared as testimony to his wise and benign reign.

Philosophical Influences

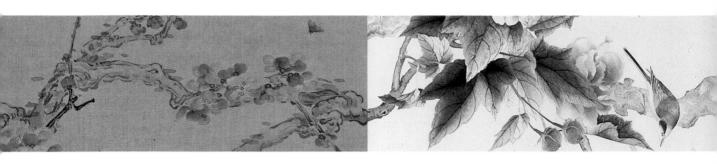

As noted earlier, the theories essential to the practice of medicine were part of the overall Chinese view of the world; in other words, philosophy. The most inherent and widely known of these are the theories of Yin Yang and the Five Elements, which spring from the underlying concept of Tao. (We shall be looking at the actual theories themselves in depth in Part Two.)

The Tao, usually translated as the Way, is an explanation of how the universe came into being, how the forces at work in the universe interplay, and how people can harmonize with nature by adhering to the Tao. It is easy to understand how the ancient Chinese, who were an agriculture-based society, would have seen the cycles and forces at work in nature and developed a system of beliefs and behavior that mirrored the processes they observed in nature itself. Proof of someone's adherence to the Tao was said to be seen in their state of health and longevity; many ancient Chinese texts make reference to the sages of times past who had lived for well over a hundred years. The formalization of this philosophy of "going with the flow" took place with the development of Taoism, and the writing of the Tao Te Ching by Lao Tzu around the sixth century B.C.E. However, the concepts of Tao and Yin Yang had been part of the Chinese psyche for centuries prior to this.

The earliest recorded reference to Yin Yang is in the I Ching, the Book of Changes. Traditionally the original trigrams described in the I Ching are said to have been discovered by Fu Hsi (the Chinese equivalent of Adam) drawn on the back of a tortoise that crawled out of the Yellow River. Legend puts this

ABOVE *Examples of Chinese and Japanese art, showing the freer Taoist influence in Chinese art (left), and the more formal realism of the Japanese (right).*

date at around 5000 B.C.E. Dates of commentaries are somewhat more certain: those of King Wen and his son the Duke of Chu around 1144 B.C.E., and one by Confucius (551–479 B.C.E.). The high point in I Ching studies was reached during the Han Dynasty, at which time the separate theories of medicine from the North and South of China were being joined together to form a comprehensive whole.

Five Element theory (often translated as Five Phases or Five Transformations) was developed later than Yin Yang, initially as an independent theory. It had wide influence in the arts, culture, and politics. Five Element theory was merged with Yin Yang theory by Tsou Yen (c. 340–260 B.C.E.), leader of the Yin Yang philosophical school. Further classic texts such as *The Spiritual Axis: Ling She Jing, The Classic of Difficulties: Nan Jing Jiao Shi*, and *The Classic of the Pulse: Mai Jing* ensued, bringing together the accumulated knowledge, research, philosophical development, and practical experience of medical practitioners over the centuries. These and many other works form a very large body of literature on oriental medical theory and practice, which are still read, respected, and referred to as authority even today.

Oriental Medical Theory Spreads to Japan

The migration of these ideas to Japan did not commence until about the sixth century C.E. Buddhism was introduced to Japan somewhere between 538 and 552 C.E., and with it came an influx of Chinese philosophy and culture. Taoism, Buddhism, and Confucianism were the three main strands in Chinese thought, each combining and weaving together in different measure the concepts of Tao and Yin Yang. Trading and diplomatic missions increased the contact between Japan and China, and in 608 C.E. Prince Shotuku sent a delegation of Japanese students to China to learn Chinese culture and medicine. By 984 C.E. the oldest existing Japanese medical text had been written: the 30-volume Ishinho by Tamba Yasuyori.

However, the great flowering of oriental medicine took place during the Edo Period (1603–1868) as the Tokugawa Shoguns turned their backs on the European influence of the Dutch and Portuguese and fostered the development of oriental traditions. They decreed that massage was a profession that could be taken up by the blind, since their sense of touch is extra sensitive. Inevitably, since educational opportunities for the blind

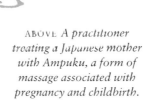

ABOVE A practitioner treating a Japanese mother with Ampuku, a form of massage associated with pregnancy and childbirth.

LEFT The elements of the Yin Yang symbol – the circular shape, the curving dividing line, and the two spots – are expressive of the inclusive philosophy of the Tao.

were restricted, the medical aspects of Anma began to be lost. Masseurs became less qualified than doctors and were therefore less highly regarded. Also, doctors were using the whole range of medical techniques with an emphasis on herbal treatment that, because of the ingestion of substances into the body, required rigorous training. Doctors and herbalists were seen as working more in the realm of medicine, while Anma massage was associated principally with relaxation and pleasure.

It is interesting to note, however, that the medical application of massage technique was retained in the area of pregnancy and childbirth, by the use of a Japanese form of abdominal treatment known as Ampuku. Ampuku is a specialized form of abdominal massage that has been used medicinally for centuries. It is effective in the treatment of many conditions but has particular application to gynecological problems and childbirth and its notable association with relaxation may well have been helpful to women in labor. This practice is noted in the chapter on "Midwifery in Japan" in *The Women* by Ploss and Bartels. A Doctor Sigen Kangawa wrote a book on obstetrics called *The San-ron* (the "Description of Birth") in 1765. Kangawa made use in obstetrics of Ampuku, a massage in that has been in use in Japan from ancient times and is said to help various maladies. He introduced it as a methodical, careful, and gentle pressure or palpation of the abdomen for the diagnosis of pregnancy, as well as for the acceleration of delivery and for the elimination of various ills of pregnant women.

2 The Development of Modern Shiatsu

The devaluation of Anma massage as a form of medical treatment continued into the early twentieth century, when there was a revival signaling the start of the modern history of Shiatsu. The catalyst for this revival was the publication in 1919 of a book entitled *Shiatsu Ho* by Tamai Tempaku. He practiced Anma, Ampuku, and Do-in, and in addition had made considerable studies in Western anatomy, physiology, and massage. It seems that his work was instrumental in stimulating further research, and influenced several practitioners whose subsequent work considerably advanced the development of Shiatsu in the forms we now know it. Notable among these were Tokujiro Namikoshi, Katsusuke Serizawa, and Shizuto Masunaga.

Since the mid-1970s and the publication in English of Toru Namikoshi's *Shiatsu Therapy: Theory and Practice* (1974), Serizawa's *Tsubo: Vital Points for Oriental Therapy* (1976), and Masunaga's *Zen Shiatsu* (1977), the therapy has expanded rapidly in the U.K., U.S.A., Europe, and Australasia.

In many countries, practitioners have joined together to form national Shiatsu Societies, which promote public awareness and seek official recognition of Shiatsu as a therapy. The European Shiatsu Society has helped to gain Shiatsu recognition as a Non-Conventional Medical discipline within the European Union. In the U.S. the original professional organization, the American Shiatsu Association, has joined with other therapies to form the A.O.B.T.A. (The American Oriental Bodywork Therapy Association). The Shiatsu Therapy Association of Australia is likewise involved with establishing support groups, organizing international conferences, and implementing the development of national standards for Shiatsu practitioners.

THREE INFLUENTIAL PRACTITIONERS

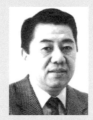

Namikoshi

Namikoshi-style Shiatsu "relies on the proper application of carefully judged pressure on specific points... to eliminate fatigue and stimulate the body's natural self-curative abilities." In Namikoshi therapy, no mention is made of energy (Ki) or meridians. Namikoshi's major contribution was to establish Shiatsu as an officially recognized therapy in Japan.

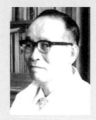

Serizawa

Serizawa's work is specifically concerned with the therapeutic properties of individual points (tsubo) and the techniques that can be applied to them, depending on the nature of the problem. While basing his research on oriental medicine, he believes the scientific explanation of the meridian systems and tsubo "as nerve reflex action is the most satisfactory."

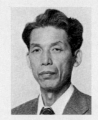

Masunaga

Masunaga has had more influence on Shiatsu outside Japan than any other teacher. His comprehensive method, known as Zen Shiatsu, emphasizes the use of meridians and includes an extended meridian system, a detailed form of diagnosis through abdominal palpation, and a specific theory explaining imbalance within the body and mind.

Namikoshi-style Shiatsu

Namikoshi initially used rubbing and pressing techniques to help his mother, who was afflicted with arthritis. He trained in Anma technique, but continued to develop his own method and in 1925 opened the Shiatsu Institute of Therapy in Hokkaido. By 1940 he had transferred his center to Tokyo, where he established the Japan Shiatsu Institute. In 1955 Shiatsu was legally approved as part of Anma massage, and the Japan Shiatsu School was licensed by the Japanese Minister of Health and Welfare two years later. Shiatsu was finally recognized as a therapy in its own right as distinct from Anma and Western (Swedish) massage in 1964. Quite when the term Shiatsu was actually coined is not recorded in any written text, but it is undoubtedly a modern word used to distinguish the form from Anma and Ampuku.

Namikoshi's major contribution was the gaining of official recognition for Shiatsu, the establishment of a training school, and his extensive teaching, which spread information about Shiatsu throughout Japan and to the U.S.A. It is perhaps ironic that in his eagerness to have Shiatsu accepted by the Western scientific mind, Namikoshi removed all mention of meridians, energy, and traditional theory from his work, and thus his style of practice tends to appeal less to the modern generation of bodywork students who are actively seeking a subtle, even spiritual, aspect to bring to their work.

Tokujiro Namikoshi's approach has been continued by his son Toru Namikoshi who spent seven years teaching Shiatsu in the United States and Europe, and set down a comprehensive guide to this style in his book *The Complete Book of Shiatsu Therapy*. The techniques used in this form of Shiatsu are very physical and symptomatic, working largely on neuromuscular points and around areas of pain.

The theoretical basis of Namikoshi-style Shiatsu depends upon detailed knowledge of the muscular, skeletal, nervous, and endocrine systems, in short a very Western approach, while the overall view on good health is somewhat more traditional and includes advice on good diet, elimination, exercise, and laughter.

Although Shiatsu is still practiced in Japan, much of its development in terms of research, recognition of its therapeutic benefits, and the expansion of knowledge and application of theory is currently taking place in Western countries.

BELOW *Namikoshi-style Shiatsu works primarily on the physical level.*

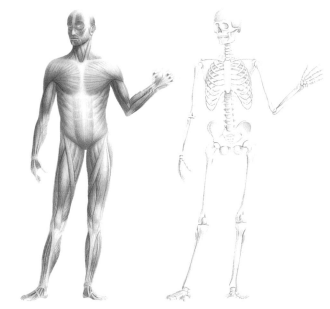

Muscular system

Skeletal system

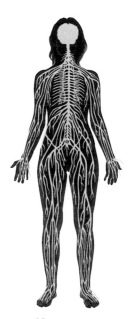

Nervous system

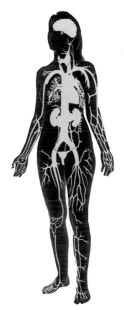

Endocrine system

Tsubo Therapy

Katsusuke Serizawa concentrated his research into the nature and effects of the tsubo; that is, the points themselves. Using the traditional concepts of oriental medicine he studied the location and functions of the tsubo found on the meridians, and utilizing modern electrical methods of measurement he tested the meridians and their tsubo to prove their existence scientifically. In recognition of this important experimental research he was awarded a Doctor of Medicine degree in 1961. Tsubo Therapy, as Serizawa calls his method of treatment, concentrates very much on the therapeutic qualities of the points and can use massage, pressure, acupuncture, moxa, or any of the more modern stimulating gadgets that are currently on the market. This is a little different in approach from the standard form of Shiatsu, but a derivation of this style, Acupressure Shiatsu, is practiced in the U.S. utilizing various acupuncture classifications of points.

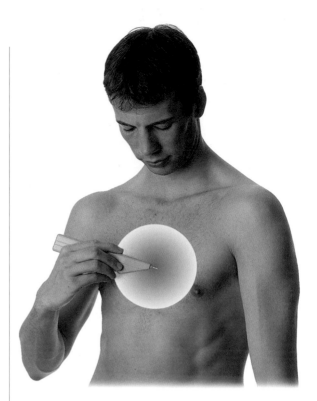

ABOVE *Self-stimulation using a battery-operated electronic device for activating tsubos.*

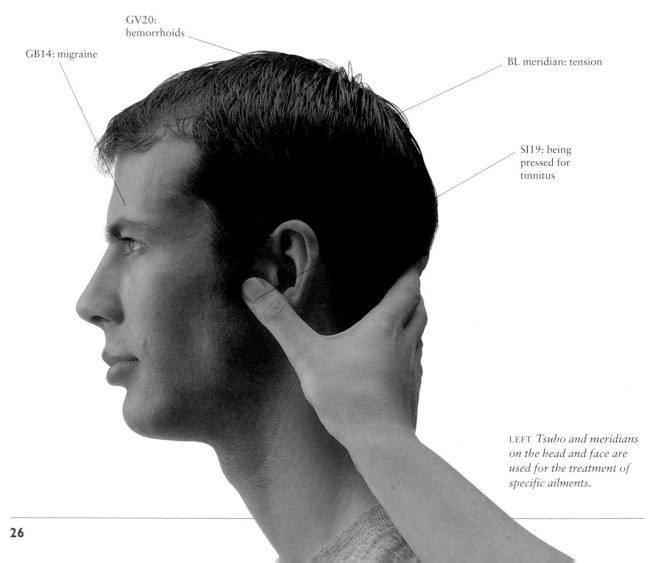

GV20: hemorrhoids

GB14: migraine

BL meridian: tension

SI19: being pressed for tinnitus

LEFT *Tsubo and meridians on the head and face are used for the treatment of specific ailments.*

Other Forms and Styles of Shiatsu

Shiatsu, like many other disciplines, has its own particular history, which has led different individuals to focus upon different aspects of the overall therapy. Several distinctive styles have been given specific names denoting their theoretical approach or their originator. We have already mentioned Namikoshi style, Zen Shiatsu, and Acupressure Shiatsu or Tsubo Therapy. In addition to these, the other forms generally acknowledged are Macrobiotic Shiatsu, which incorporates Barefoot Shiatsu and integrates the use of traditional meridians with the dietary and lifestyle theories of George Ohsawa, Michio Kushi, and Shizuko Yamamoto. Ohashiatsu is the method used by Wataru Ohashi, incorporating aspects of Zen Shiatsu and Namikoshi style with the use of traditional meridians. Five Element Shiatsu is similar in theory and methodology to Five Element Acupuncture, using the dynamic of the Five Elements and a classification of points according to their element influence: this form is practiced mostly in the U.S. Nippon Shiatsu is again an American designation, basically comprising Namikoshi's method with knowledge of the traditional meridians. As well as these distinctive styles, some Shiatsu practitioners have been greatly influenced by Traditional Chinese Medicine (T.C.M.), a specific theory of acupuncture and herbalism. They tend to use T.C.M. as a theoretical model, although their actual technique is usually closer to Zen or Namikoshi Shiatsu than to modern Chinese massage, Tui-Na.

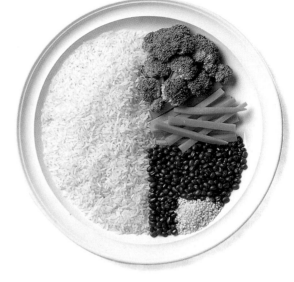

ABOVE *Macrobiotic Shiatsu incorporates dietary strictures involving the consumption of whole grains, raw vegetables, and fruit.*

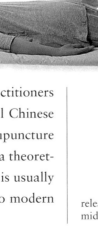

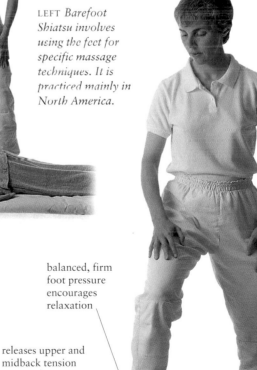

LEFT *Barefoot Shiatsu involves using the feet for specific massage techniques. It is practiced mainly in North America.*

balanced, firm foot pressure encourages relaxation

releases upper and midback tension

RIGHT *By moving from hara and using released body weight, the practitioner can work effectively on chronically tight muscles.*

Zen Shiatsu

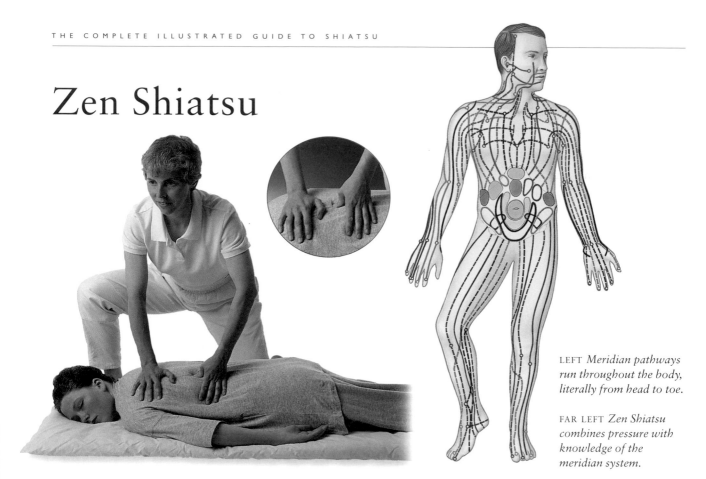

LEFT *Meridian pathways run throughout the body, literally from head to toe.*

FAR LEFT *Zen Shiatsu combines pressure with knowledge of the meridian system.*

The key figure in the development of Shiatsu in the later part of the twentieth century was Shizuto Masunaga. Where Namikoshi places no reliance on the meridian system, Masunaga brought Shiatsu firmly back into the realms of traditional oriental theory. He pioneered a system, usually referred to as Zen Shiatsu, which seeks to discover which of the "life aspects" described by the meridian functions is disturbed, and uses a specific theory of energy balance (known as kyo-jitsu theory) to interpret this. Masunaga extended the acupuncture meridians to form a more complex network of traditional and "supplementary" meridians that give the practitioner increased scope to work creatively with the body's energy. He also developed a detailed and specific form of abdominal diagnosis.

COMPARISON OF ZEN SHIATSU WITH OTHER METHODS

Zen	Other techniques
Uses relaxed weight rather than muscle strength resulting in greater penetration and sensitivity.	May tend to recommend certain number of pounds of pressure.
Requires direction of pressure to be perpendicular (at 90° to the body) to allow effective access to the body's Ki.	May use vibration and rotation as well as stationary pressure
Always uses two hands on the body, usually a quieter "mother" hand and a more active working hand.	May use only one hand on the body, or both thumbs on one point.
Works the whole length of the imbalanced meridian in order to reintegrate it into the body's Ki flow.	Work specific points only, or parts of meridians affected by imbalance.
Emphasizes the relaxation and posture of the giver to increase effectiveness and sensitivity.	May place variable importance on posture and relaxation.

Common Strands within Shiatsu

From the previous paragraphs we may have the impression that Shiatsu is very much divided, but in fact there is a common core of technique running through all approaches that is summed up in the therapy's name, "Shiatsu," which means "finger pressure." Shiatsu is about pressure on the body; whether the practitioner describes his or her theoretical basis in terms of meridians and tsubo or trigger/neuromuscular points, the fact remains that Shiatsu involves pressing, rubbing, and stretching the body in order to

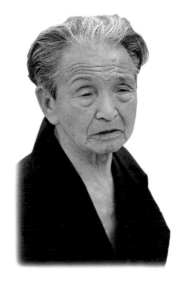

ABOVE *Shiatsu has remained popular with the older generation in Japan.*

revitalize it. For this reason we find that generally practitioners and students can use more than one approach quite compatibly within their treatment. Indeed, in Great Britain the regulatory organization for Shiatsu, the Shiatsu Society, actively encourages cross-fertilization of ideas and therapeutic approaches by requiring practitioners who wish to go onto its professional register to have studied more than one style of Shiatsu. This is to give students an understanding of other ways of working, and thus to avoid the rifts that have from time to time dogged the progress of other therapies.

In Japan, Shiatsu remains popular with the older generation, who have retained the more traditional ways, while younger people seem to

prefer Western medicine. However, forms of Shiatsu are widely taught by the martial arts schools as the healing aspect of their disciplines. In contrast, Shiatsu is growing in popularity in Great Britain, the U.S., parts of Europe, and Australasia, where people are looking for a holistic way of bodywork that is able to incorporate a strong spiritual or esoteric element.

Shiatsu is a growing and developing discipline. Far from being trapped in the past or fossilized into set techniques, it is continuing to progress and push back the boundaries of our understanding of Ki energy and our ability to direct Ki for healing in the body. While acknowledging and respecting our ancient historical roots and the great teachers of the past, we can move forward using all kinds of methodologies, from the esoteric to the scientific, to continue the development of Shiatsu as a living, dynamic therapy.

RIGHT *A traditional Japanese kendo class. Shiatsu practitioners encourage contacts with other philosophical disciplines.*

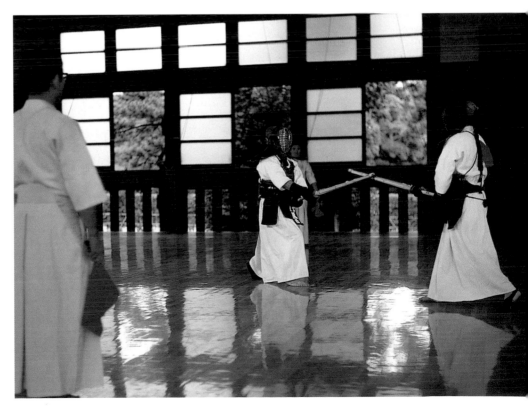

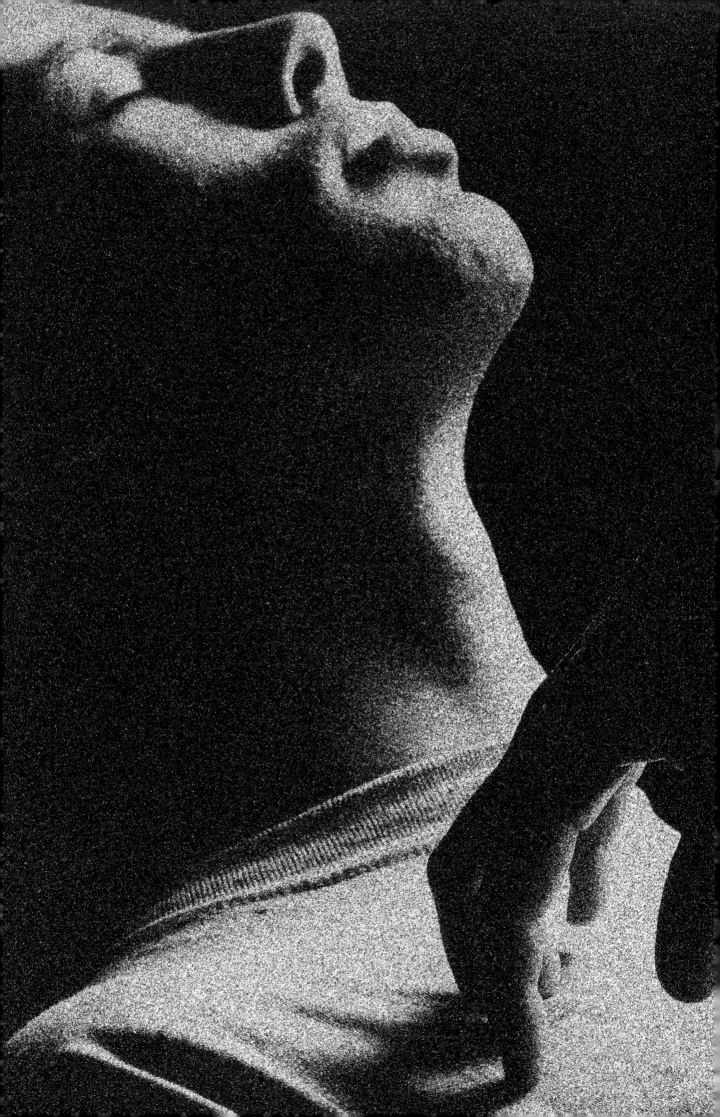

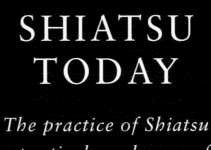

SHIATSU
TODAY

The practice of Shiatsu has particular relevance for modern life, with its holistic approach to healing mind and body.

1 Zen Shiatsu and Today's World

It is interesting that of all the styles and approaches to Shiatsu, the one that has gained most acceptance in the Western world is Masunaga's Zen Shiatsu. The reasons for this are many and varied and may be the result, in no small part, of the enthusiastic dissemination of his work in the U.S. and Europe by such inspiring teachers as Pauline Sasaki and Clifford Andrews.

Zen Shiatsu is, by its intrinsically Zen nature, a form of healing that addresses the receiver now, in this moment of need. Let us take an example of a client arriving for treatment with chronic headaches. Zen Shiatsu recognizes that the practitioner has to deal with her feelings today of, let us say, hurt and lack of worth at a colleague's ill-timed words, before getting down to strategies and techniques for reducing the long-term problem. The immediate upset emotions and accompanying mental attitude ("I work so hard and do so much for everyone else, how could she say that to me?") have disturbed her energetic system out of its usual pattern. By choosing to work on the meridian that relates most to this particular emotional upset, the practitioner can address the temporary disturbance and help the client work through it, using the medium of the body's energetic structure. Part way through the session our client gives a big sigh and wriggles her body. This is a signal to the practitioner that an energetic change has occurred; the energetic diagnosis is taken again and the practitioner notes a change in the meridian that was showing the most need or deficiency.

It is this sensitivity to changing Ki patterns, even within one treatment, that gives Zen Shiatsu its power and immediacy. Or to put it another way, in such a scenario the practitioner is clearly treating *the person* rather than the condition. This very human and immediate attitude is not common in everyday life, where we often feel we are "just another number," and even though some institutions and sectors of modern society do strive toward being "person-centered," in practice this may not be the experience of the client or receiver.

Addressing emotions, attitudes, and thought patterns, as well as physical symptoms, is built into the Zen Shiatsu system because it is a system focused on the movement of Ki within the meridian structure. Masunaga had extensive knowledge of traditional oriental medicine, but coupled this with his studies in psychology and an interest in the dynamics of Ki energy. It is the psychological aspect that integrates the whole of Masunaga's system and makes sense of the relationship between physical symptoms and the psycho-emotional state.

LEFT *Many of the problems Shiatsu treats arise in the workplace, either from posture or out of emotional situations.*

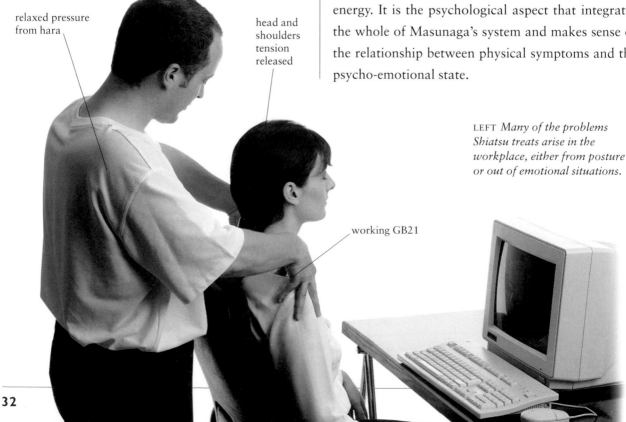

relaxed pressure from hara

head and shoulders tension released

working GB21

LOOKING BEHIND THE PROBLEM

By focusing on the "kyo," the hidden or underlying cause of disease, Zen Shiatsu can be a medium for creating long-term changes where perhaps a more symptomatic approach, dealing with the excess or jitsu meridian imbalance (see p. 80), would not have such a profound effect. It is so easy in our modern, pressured world to look at the obvious problem and just fix that so that we can rush on to the next activity or project, without looking at what may be behind it. With its emphasis on which meridian function is under-active and its relationship to the conse-quent overactive meridian, Zen Shiatsu encourages people to be more aware of their overall pat-terns and encourages them to take responsibility for their own health. The attitude of our client then changes from "Cure my headaches," to "Why do I get headaches? What is it about my energetic makeup, my thought patterns, and attitudes that is creating this chronic condition? Is it my work practices or posture? Is it hormonally based?"

These questions can be answered using meridian theory and by making the client aware of the correspon-dences between the physical and psycho-emotional aspects of the meridians. This kind of reasoning can often make a lot of sense and allows people to see how everyday events can affect health in a definite manner. The practitioner, as well as administering Shiatsu, would suggest self-help exercises for balancing Ki in the affected meridians, would give tsubo indications for everyday use, both preventively and during a headache, and might work out assertiveness strategies or suggest an appoint-ment with a counselor to look at the thought patterns that are part of the problem. Often a small shift in personal attitude or daily habits can do much to break long-term patterns.

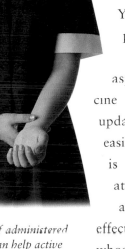

ABOVE *Self administered Shiatsu can help active workers such as nurses ease the aches and pains of their busy schedules.*

Conventional medicine, and even some of the alternative therapies that do not emphasize the underlying cause, would probably prescribe medica-tion for the headaches themselves. This might be effective in getting rid of each individual pain attack, but would not address the "why" of the condition.

A NONINTRUSIVE INTEGRATED SYSTEM

In summary, Masunaga's whole method, theory, diagnosis, and treatment is a comprehensive and integrated system, specifically designed for practitioners using touch and pressure. Firmly based on Masunaga's extensive research into and knowledge of traditional ori-ental medicine, the theoretical aspect of Zen Shiatsu is derived from Yin Yang and Five Element theory (see pp. 50 and 54). However, some of the more obscure and esoteric aspects of traditional oriental medi-cine are explained in a somewhat updated fashion, making them more easily accessible to the Western mind. It is interesting that Shiatsu is now attracting medical doctors, nurses, and physiotherapists as being an effective and all-encompassing therapy, whose theory is not incompatible with (although different from) modern science. In fact, at the time of writing, a doctor studying at the Glasgow School of Shiatsu in Scotland has said she has rarely found a Shiatsu meridian diagnosis to be inaccurate.

Being a nonintrusive therapy, Shiatsu as a whole is finding favor with many people. The emphasis in Zen Shiatsu on working on the underlying causes of health problems, coupled with its cohesive theory of emotional and psychological correspondences with the physical, makes it particularly applicable to today's world. Zen Shiatsu strikes a chord with the ever-increasing number of people who are seeking a sense of wholeness in their lives, rather than the sim-plistic "magic pill" to cure their ills.

The Session Itself

The format of a Shiatsu session will vary according-ing to the degree of experience and expertise of the practitioner. Beginners tend to follow a "form" in which all the meridians are generally stimulated, producing an overall relaxing effect. An experienced professional practitioner generally begins a series of treatments only after taking a detailed case history from the patient. By palpating the abdomen (known in Japanese as the hara) and the back, and possibly by feeling the pulses, the patient's energetic state can be assessed. From the information gained, the practitioner may choose to work on one, two, or more meridians, using stretches to open the body before stimulating the points. The techniques used depend entirely upon the patient's energetic state and needs.

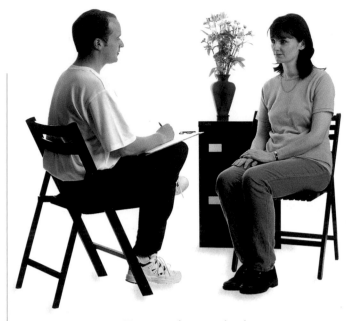

ABOVE *Treatment begins only after detailed questioning of the patient's background and symptoms.*

More dynamic moves such as rocking, shaking, and stretching help to disperse and move blocked Ki. Long, deep thumb pressure on specific points or palming a meridian helps to draw Ki to areas of weakness and emptiness. When working on large or heavily muscled people, the practitioner may make extensive use of elbows, knees, and feet. This is in order to be more effective in contacting the Ki. It also prevents the practitioner from becoming overtired when moving a large body about. When working on children, babies, or very elderly patients, pressure is usually very light, and some practitioners even work on them at the etheric level; that is, above the body but within the body's energetic field, where physical pressure is inappropriate.

No two Shiatsu sessions are ever alike. The order of work, the choice of meridians to be stimulated, and the areas on which to concentrate always change with the receiver's

LEFT *Handwritten case notes made by an experienced practitioner.*

NAME Jeff Cartwright

ADDRESS South Hourat, Dalry

TELEPHONE NUMBER Home Kil 889   Work

OCCUPATION Engineer (retired)   Over/Under/OK

HEIGHT 5ft 4ins   **WEIGHT** 12 stone

DATE OF BIRTH 6-5-25   **TIME OF BIRTH**

MARITAL STATUS Married/Single/Divorced/Separated   **REFERRED BY** Daughter

NUMBER OF CHILDREN 3

CURRENT PROBLEMS

When and how sickness occurred left leg pain originating in knee following fall. Pain mostly on side of knee, on bad days, left buttock and thigh affected

Medication being taken Ibuprofen based cream

Sleep pattern
☒ Normal ☐ Insomnia ☐ Sleeps too much ☐ Lots of dreams ☐ Easily awakened
☐ Doesn't feel sleepy ☐ Other

Headaches
☐ None ☐ Heavy feeling ☐ Dizzy ☐ Faints when stands up
☐ Like blow on head ☒ Nausea
Location of headaches Migraine at night. Frontal and left side

Bowel movements
☐ regular ☐ hard ☐ soft ☒ flatulence ☐ constipation ☐ diarrhea
how many times per day 1 or more ☐ constantly going

Urine
☒ regular ☐ lots ☐ little
☐ night time (how much) 1 or more **how many times per day** History of prostate enlargement ☐ vomit ☐ indigestion

Stomach
☒ normal ☐ can't eat ☒ heartburn ☐ belching ☐ right
When it hurts, where does it hurt? ☐ side ☐ left
☐ lower
☐ upper

conditions. This makes Shiatsu stimulating to give as well as to receive. Here the practitioner's creativity comes into play, blending intuition and knowledge of theory in order to construct a complete and appropriate session for that patient at that time. So each Shiatsu session is a unique event.

Within each session there is a balance between general work, with mobilization and stretches, and specific work on certain meridians. By concentrating on a particular meridian and its associated functions, the practitioner can focus the receiver's self-healing abilities where they are most needed to get to the heart of the problem – an important point when working on someone with very low energy.

Unlike acupuncture or acupressure massage, where the therapist concentrates on a few specific points, in Shiatsu the whole of an imbalanced meridian (or long stretches of it) are stimulated. There is an emphasis on normalizing the muscles and joints around the meridian as well as regulating the Ki in that particular channel. While making use of the traditional acupuncture points, known in Japanese as tsubo, Shiatsu also recognizes that Ki may be disturbed anywhere along a meridian. Practitioners therefore work all along the meridians using intuition and developed sensitivity in the hands to locate imbalance points and bring their energy to the same level as the rest of the meridian. Very often this involves long and slow holding with the degree of pressure depending on the feel of the tsubo. This holding of points is characteristic of Shiatsu, often making it look as though nothing is happening in the treatment. However, the patient will have an intense consciousness of being connected to that point, while at a physiological level the static pressure allows chronically tight muscles to release. Since emotions, old thoughts, and memories can be locked up in the soft tissues of the body,

ABOVE *The practitioner will continue to take notes to chart progress at each session.*

Shiatsu practitioners often find that patients experience emotional release during treatment. In the long term this can help in dealing with deep-seated psycho-emotional conditions.

During the session the practitioner generally works all over the body: arms, legs, back, abdomen, neck, and head. This overall treatment again gives the patient the sense of being put back in touch with the whole body, not just the part that may be the current problem. Connecting up the parts draws the patient's attention to the relationships between parts of the physical body and the mind, something that is normally overlooked.

The Effects of Treatment

At the end of the treatment the patient is left to rest for a little while. In fact people often fall asleep during the session so a few minutes of recovery time are therefore essential before "coming back to the here and now." After treatment the patient usually feels very relaxed, with a sense of well-being and peace. Sometimes there is also a feeling of invigoration, increased "get up and go." Both of these reactions can be put down to the deep energetic effect of the work. Occasionally a new patient may have "healing reactions" after the first few sessions. These occur when toxins have been released during the treatment, and as these work out through the body there may be symptoms such as headache, stiffness, stomach upsets or diarrhea, desire to urinate frequently, or lethargy. Such symptoms are transitory and soon pass, usually in 12 hours at most. Drinking plenty of spring water and resting will help, as well as asking the practitioner for advice and reassurance if you are at all worried.

Emotional releases may take longer to work through, and indeed, over the course of a number of treatments, deep-seated emotional patterns or memories involving past emotions may be uncovered. These can have profound effects on the patient's life. In such cases, extra contact between sessions may be necessary to talk through the reactions to treatment and to look at these in the perspective of energy dynamics and meridian function.

While working meridians and specific points helps to regulate the energetic level, pressure also has the physical effect of stimulating the circulatory, lymphatic, and hormonal systems. This pressure also regulates the activity of both divisions of the autonomic nervous system and releases toxins.

These all help to activate the body's self-healing mechanisms. Shiatsu practitioners acknowledge that the healing that takes place during a session is largely due to the stimulation of the patient's self-healing abilities. The practitioner is seen as a catalyst who draws attention to certain aspects of the body, mind, or spirit that are not functioning properly. It is not uncommon for patients to say after a session: "I didn't know that that point hurt (was tight, or needed to be touched) until you pressed it." We are so often "out of touch" with our bodies and our needs: the caring and compassionate contact between practitioner and patient in Shiatsu can do much to reintroduce ourselves to our bodies and in so doing can help to ease any feelings of alienation and lack of communication with others.

LEFT *After treatment, people may notice postural changes – being more upright and able to "look the world in the eye."*

TOXINS

Toxins can accumulate in cells throughout the body because of inappropriate diet, excess alcohol, or drugs, or the after-effects of exercise. Cramp may result from the presence of lactic acid in the muscles if there has been insufficient cellular activity to "burn through" the glucose used as fuel in muscular activity.

Practicalities

Shiatsu is very practical in that very little equipment is required. It is almost always practiced on the floor, on a thin Japanese cotton futon or mattress. This practice has arisen through tradition; in Japan there is very little space in dwellings and people sleep on futons that can be rolled up during the day, leaving the living space clear. However, there are other practical considerations: being at floor level means the practitioner can use body weight rather than muscle power to apply pressure. This is much more comfortable to receive, and certainly less tiring on the practitioner. Shiatsu can also be given in a sitting position on a chair, or lying on the side – useful for pregnant women and people with certain back or chest conditions. All these factors make it very easy to give Shiatsu wherever you are; at home, in the office, even on the beach! Of course, professional treatment with a qualified practitioner takes place in a more formal treatment room, which is light, airy, and comfortably warm. Some practitioners go out of their way to create a harmonious atmosphere in the room, so that the session is a complete experience involving all five senses, somewhat like experiencing a Japanese tea ceremony.

Shiatsu is performed through light clothing – a cotton sweatsuit or similar garment is ideal. Paradoxically, working through clothes enables the practitioner to concentrate on the feel of the tsubo rather than being distracted by looking. It is interesting to note that in Japan Shiatsu is one of the recognized professions for the blind, whose sense of touch can be so finely developed.

ABOVE *Hunching the shoulders and dropping the head is not only bad for the back but impedes the energy system.*

RIGHT *Shiatsu is usually more comfortable and easier to apply with the patient lying on the floor.*

THE PATIENT'S PREPARATION

Do

- wear loose clothing such as a sweatsuit that will keep you warm, as the metabolic rate usually slows, leading to feeling cold.
- allow enough time so that you are not arriving in a hurry, or rushing away afterward.
- have a snack about an hour before the session so you are neither full nor hungry.
- rest afterward; make the rest of the day a relaxing one.
- drink plenty of spring water to flush out any toxins released.
- if being treated at home, ensure that the room is warm and quiet, and free from disturbances.

Don't

- drink alcohol on the day of treatment.
- eat large or heavy meals.
- exercise more than normal.
- take an excessively hot bath.
- wear perfume, aftershave, or other cosmetics (such as deodorant), since these can mask your own smell, which may be used in diagnosis.

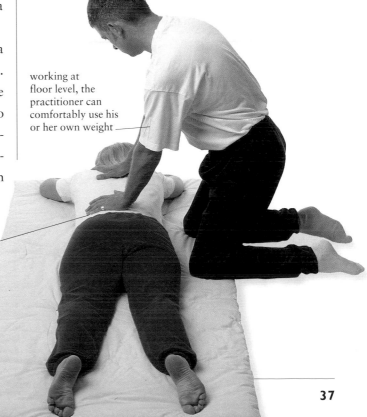

working at floor level, the practitioner can comfortably use his or her own weight

pressure is applied through the clothing

the patient usually lies on a futon or mattress

2 Shiatsu and Other Therapies

Where does Shiatsu stand in relation to other therapies? I feel that Shiatsu occupies an area of middle ground between acupuncture, massage, and healing, because it shares certain essential aspects with all three of these disciplines. In addition, Shiatsu has strong similarities and links with both reflexology and yoga. The combination of these forms a unique and powerful tool for healing and change. Shiatsu has a very distinctive feel that is unlike other forms of bodywork, and this often comes as a surprise to people accustomed to experiencing massage, aromatherapy, or reflexology.

Let us look at the common elements and the differences between Shiatsu, massage, healing, acupuncture, reflexology, and yoga.

Massage

Massage and Shiatsu share many aspects: the warm and compassionate touch of another human being, encouraging the body to let go and relax. Both forms work on the physical site of pain or stiffness and can release emotional disturbances. Western massage theory and a knowledge of physiology can be used to explain the mechanisms of physical dysfunction. Shiatsu, on the other hand, also enjoys the more poetic, yet commonsense, explanation embodied in oriental medical theory to give the patient an overall view of the condition. Where Shiatsu differs from most forms of massage, except for the obvious aspects mentioned earlier, such as being performed through clothing, is in its use of manipulation and stretches.

By manipulation I do not necessarily mean the adjustment of bones, as in osteopathy or chiropractic. Manipulation in Shiatsu is the use of passive rotations and stretches, for example, picking up the knee and lower leg of a patient lying face upward and making a wide circle to mobilize and stretch the hip joint. This standard physiotherapy technique gives a good guide to the patient's overall level of relaxation. The patient who cannot relax sufficiently to allow the

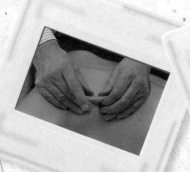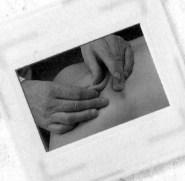

ABOVE *Massage achieves its healing effects using superficial strokes, such as rolling, that condition and tone the body's muscular structures.*

practitioner to do the rotation is often the sort of person who cannot "let go" in other aspects of life. How wide a circle can the knee make? This indicates overall flexibility. Are there any directions or parts of the rotation that are more difficult or uncomfortable? Each direction or sector of the circle can be used as a diagnostic tool to back up other observations.

Rotations are used on shoulders, wrists, ankles, fingers, and toes, and gently on the neck. Some practitioners use specific adjustment techniques where they feel there is a need. This is usually effected by putting the receiver into a stretch position and encouraging him or her to breathe through an extension of the stretch. Specific stretches are used to activate a particular area covered by a meridian, making it easier to contact and its Ki more open to change.

Healing

Healing, the laying on of hands, has a long and well-documented history. It is an ability to bring relief to others in a way that is, at present, beyond the scope of science to explain. In healing, the practitioner directs healing energy, usually in the form of light or color, to the painful or affected areas. This may be done by touching the body lightly, or by holding hands about two or three inches off the body, at the "etheric" level. The patient often has a sensation of warmth, movement, or of a breeze passing by the part being worked upon. Knowing where to place the hands and when to move to another area depends upon intuition and experience. Most of us have had our intuition educated out of us, and it takes time to learn to listen to and trust the small still voice that says "work on the right side of the neck" or "hold the liver area."

In Shiatsu, we have oriental medical theory on which to base what we do. In healing, the main energy centers or "chakras" are usually felt as the guide to which part of the body, mind, and spirit requires attention. Chakras are vortices of energy (*chakra* in Sanskrit means "wheel") that are located at seven levels, from the crown of the head down the spine to the coccyx.

The healer will begin his session by scanning the chakras and noting any differences of sensation at the different locations. The hands are then directed on or over any chakras or areas that require attention. The session finishes with a further scan and then closing the chakras down to prevent the receiver from going away feeling "spaced out" or vulnerable.

Some healers feel that their "gift" comes from God. Others develop their skills through meditation, yoga, and other activities. Most have a belief that healing comes not from the practitioner, but through him or her from some much larger entity, call it God, Spirit, Universe, or whatever. It is my belief that everyone has the ability to heal. I would say that everyone in the "caring professions," orthodox or alternative, is there because of his or her desire and ability to heal others. Technique is the framework on which to hang the cloth of intuitive healing ability.

The choice of technique or discipline depends upon the individual. Personally, I chose Shiatsu because it allows me to be very intuitive and creative, yet has a firm theoretical basis that my mind can get to grips with. However, I am also aware that we can make extensive use of the techniques of healing within Shiatsu, and certainly within my own practice I have found that these enrich my treatments considerably. Often just holding a point or area and visualizing healing energy entering can be the most powerful part of a treatment. These techniques are taught quite early on to students beginning Shiatsu and may account for the fact that beginners often have spectacular successes dealing with common ailments, with little or no knowledge of theory.

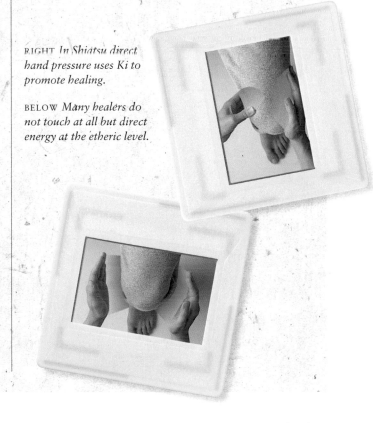

RIGHT *In Shiatsu direct hand pressure uses Ki to promote healing.*

BELOW *Many healers do not touch at all but direct energy at the etheric level.*

Acupuncture

Acupuncture and Shiatsu have common roots and share elements of theory. Whether a patient chooses acupuncture or Shiatsu as a therapy will depend upon personal preference and upon health condition. Some people like the physical closeness of Shiatsu, with its nurturing and cosseting feeling. Others like the distance of the needles. Practitioners who use both techniques tend to use acupuncture for acute, painful conditions such as arthritis, migraine, frozen shoulder, and any kind of blockage or pain. They see Shiatsu as a more nourishing and tonifying therapy that works well for chronic persistent conditions that need long work at a deeper level. Therapists who use both techniques might use acupuncture for the first part of a session to relieve acute pain and increase mobility; Shiatsu would then be used to rebalance the underlying condition, which is often due to a lack of Ki energy in certain meridians and points. Shiatsu tends to be closer in technique to Japanese acupuncture than to Chinese acupuncture.

One of the basic differences between the two disciplines is in diagnosis. In Shiatsu, because touch is involved in both the diagnosis and the work, we say that diagnosis and treatment are the same. That is, the practitioner is constantly diagnosing throughout the treatment, reassessing what he or she is feeling and modifying the session accordingly. Diagnosis is a fusion of the intuitive feelings that one gains from working on the body, and the intellectual knowledge of theory.

In acupuncture, the process is very different and much more intellectually based. The acupuncturist takes the pulses, and then decides upon a principle of treatment, choosing a formula of points that will have the specific actions needed to remedy the condition. It is rare for the treatment plan to change once the principle and points have been selected.

Japanese acupuncture tends to be more intuitive. A general principle of treatment is to find the most kyo, or deficient points, and tonify them. This may involve the use of the theory of Five Elements to tone up certain points, or it may involve palpating each meridian and quickly needling each deficient point. It is interesting to note that in Japan all acupuncturists learn Shiatsu as part of their training. It is used as a medium for teaching acupuncture, helping students to "get in touch with the Ki."

Perhaps the difference between Shiatsu and acupuncture could be summarized by saying that Shiatsu works physically on the whole body by stimulating Ki along the length of the meridians. The acupuncturist, on the other hand, looks at the whole body and then, using the theory of action of points, decides which recipe of points will most affect the whole. To quote a patient, Shiatsu gives the feeling of "being done all over."

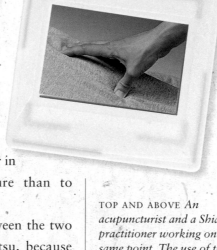

TOP AND ABOVE *An acupuncturist and a Shiatsu practitioner working on the same point. The use of the hands in Shiatsu has a more intimate feel to it than the application of needles.*

Reflexology

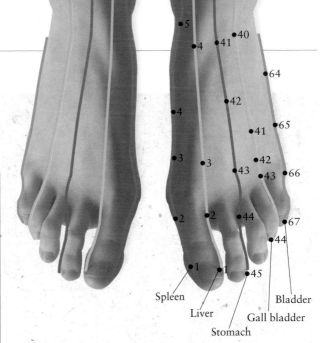

Reflexology and Shiatsu share certain similarities of technique and theory in that both utilize pressure on the body and use the idea that the internal organs can be affected by stimulation of reflex areas or points distant from the organs themselves. In reflexology, the feet are regarded as a microcosm of the whole body, with certain areas mapped out on the sole and top of the foot corresponding to organs, limbs, glands, senses, and general functions such as circulation or speech. Because of the rich supply of nerves in the feet, pressure on a precise reflex area can have an effect elsewhere in the body via the pathways of the nervous system.

Some reflexologists call their work "Zone Therapy." This divides the body longitudinally into ten zones, which correspond to five zones on each foot. Pain located in the body will then be treated by pressure on the corresponding sensitive area on the foot on that side of the body. The reflex areas map is more complex, with the toes representing the head and brain functions, the spine being found along the inside arch of both feet, and the thoracic, abdominal, and pelvic

ABOVE *For Shiatsu practitioners, the feet mark the limits of certain meridians, with several useful tsubo.*

organs being located at the ball, arch, and heel of the foot, respectively. These areas are different from the meridians of acupuncture and in some cases specific points relate to completely different organs. For example, the solar plexus area, found centrally and below the foot in reflexology, is the acupuncture point for the beginning of the Kidney meridian. (KD1 – Bubbling Spring; see p. 163.)

Both reflexology and Shiatsu rely upon the sensitivity of the practitioner's hands to effect treatment, but otherwise technique is fairly different. The standard reflexology "rotating thumb technique" is never used in Shiatsu.

BELOW *Like Shiatsu and acupuncture, reflexology uses meridian theory focusing on meridian terminals in the feet and toes.*

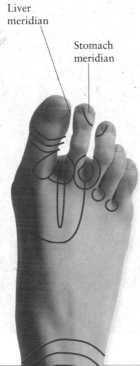

Liver meridian

Stomach meridian

Spleen/Pancreas meridian

MERIDIANS IN REFLEXOLOGY

Some modern reflexologists feel that by combining knowledge of reflexology techniques with the meridian theories of oriental medicine, they have an additional diagnostic tool, from which they can gain further insight into the nature of their patient's imbalance. On the six meridians running through the feet (SP/ST, LV/GB, KD/BL), there are many particularly useful points with a wide range of actions. Knowledge and use of these can enhance the reflexology treatment.

Yoga

Yoga must be the oldest therapeutic exercise system known to humankind. Its aim is the expansion of our human consciousness so that universal consciousness is ultimately achieved. Yoga is thus a discipline that encompasses the development of a healthy body, quiet mind, and expanded spirit. To the dedicated it becomes a spiritual pathway involving consciousness within all everyday activities, as well as during time taken in meditation and practice of poses.

The history of yoga dates back thousands of years, and the ancient yogic texts show that extremely detailed knowledge of the body's energetic entity has been with us for much of this time. Energy, called *prana* (which means "the breath" in Sanskrit), was seen to flow throughout the body in *nadis*, or channels, and interact with the chakras – seven wheels or vortices of energy which are located down the spine from crown to coccyx. The foundation of Hatha (physical) yoga is the practice of postures (*asanas*) that open the body and iron out energetic blockages within it. Breathing techniques (*pranayama*) and meditation quieten the mind. These practices allow energies to refine through the chakra system, facilitating spiritual development.

COMBINING SPIRITUAL WITH PHYSICAL

Many people attending yoga classes are unaware of the spiritual aims but enjoy the stretching and strengthening that physical yoga offers. Seen in meridian terms, the poses can stimulate Ki flow through the meridians, thus helping to either unblock or activate the functioning of the internal organs. It is very interesting to note the similarities between many yoga postures and the Shiatsu meridian stretch positions used during treatment. In my Shiatsu school, I have trained several yoga teachers and they often comment on the therapeutic effects of certain poses and how they relate to meridians. In fact someone once described Shiatsu as being "like having yoga done to you!"

ABOVE *Achieving bodily balance in standing postures is an important aspect of yoga.*

In a well-balanced yoga session or class, there will be an initial warming up sequence, followed by a series of postures to open the body and stretch all parts. Usually there is a balance between standing and floor poses, front and back bends, side twists, and inverted poses. The session will end with more gentle warming down work and a period of breathing exercises, meditation, and then rest, to allow the body, mind, and spirit to recover. Although it may seem static and not very outwardly energetic, yoga can in fact be quite strenuous and can leave you feeling pleasantly tired, with a feeling of inner peace. A Shiatsu treatment may follow a similar pattern with quieter work initially as the practitioner familiarizes him- or herself with the receiver's Ki state. More detailed techniques to rebalance

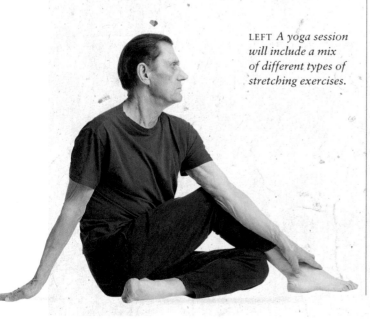

LEFT *A yoga session will include a mix of different types of stretching exercises.*

specific areas and meridians follow, possibly using stretches and different positions (such as face downward, or side lying). The end of the session usually involves gentle work, often on the face or feet, and then the receiver is left to rest to allow the Ki to settle into its new pattern.

Of course, yoga is essentially a solitary activity, being as it is a form of personal development, although classes may be useful in providing motivation and the companionship of like-minded people. Shiatsu, on the other hand, also has its own self-development aspects, but these are practiced in relation to another person. Where yoga practitioners may gauge their progress by the facility with which they can hold a particular pose, Shiatsu practitioners notice developments in terms of sensitivity to the receiver's Ki, accuracy of diagnosis, and beneficial effects of the treatment. Both are seeking to be "in tune" with universal energies, but the mode of attainment is different.

BELOW As in yoga, stretching is an important part of Shiatsu, but in it the practitioner will use touch to be aware of the receiver's Ki.

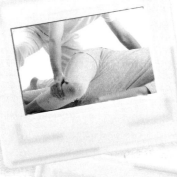

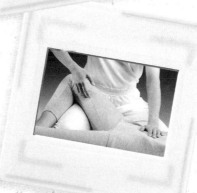

MAKKO-HO AND YOGA

In order to regulate their own Ki, Shiatsu practitioners and students often practice a series of yoga-like exercises known as the "Makko-ho" stretches (see p. 148). These movements were developed by a Mr. Makko in Japan and each one not only stretches a pair of meridians but also expresses the psychological attitude behind them. For example, the stretch for Kidney and Bladder involves sitting on the floor, feet outstretched in front, and then bending forward toward the feet. The back is therefore stretched (the location of the Bladder meridian and the supplementary Kidney meridian – the Zen Shiatsu extension). In addition, these meridians govern the nervous system, impetus, and "going forward in life," all of which is symbolized in the forward stretching pose. The emphasis in working the Makko-ho is somewhat different from the attitude in yoga. Where yoga tends to be very precise about angles and which muscles are involved, the Makko-ho are done on the basis of relaxing into the stretch, and therefore the feel is quite different. Doing these six exercises is an excellent way of working all the meridians in a relatively short time.

Energy is consciously used in both Shiatsu and yoga at advanced levels: energy flow is encouraged, and the consequent psycho-emotional and spiritual benefits are acknowledged. As systems of personal development, both are very compatible and mutually supportive. Yoga can form the basis of increased knowledge of one's own Ki, and Shiatsu can allow one to apply that knowledge through helping others to become more aware of their own Ki.

To my mind, it is one of the strengths of Shiatsu that it shares elements with other disciplines and integrates them into a unique whole. Shiatsu is very compatible with other therapies and with orthodox medicine and it is common to use Shiatsu in combination with, say, herbalism, dietary therapy, or counseling.

3 Shiatsu as Self-development

One of the elements of Shiatsu not often discussed is its role in self-development. Shiatsu is not just a technique to be applied during practice hours only and left behind on leaving work for the day. To be a Shiatsu practitioner you must take the principles and theory into your heart so that Shiatsu becomes part of every aspect of your life. In the same way that yoga, meditation, or the martial arts can be a mirror in which progress through life is seen, so Shiatsu can become the focal point by which your relationship with Self, with others, and with life is measured. When the Shiatsu is going well, diagnosis becomes very clear and easy, techniques flow smoothly, intuitive feelings become certainties, and the appropriate things are said and done to promote healing. In short, good Shiatsu feels as good to give as to receive.

Students of Shiatsu often begin as patients and, finding that Shiatsu can provide a framework for self-understanding, embark upon the study of Shiatsu as a voyage of further self-discovery. The helping and healing of others through the techniques of Shiatsu is almost, in a sense, a by-product of the process of self-development. The ability to help and heal is in direct ratio to the amount of personal work the student is prepared to put in. A practitioner of Shiatsu cannot be really effective if his or her energetic state is still not balanced and harmonious. Knowing theory and technique alone is not sufficient; the Ki must be strong, and this leads to a healthy body and well-balanced outlook on life.

Self-development is implicit in the teaching and practice of Shiatsu. Classes usually begin with a period of Do-in (self-Shiatsu), stretching, or Qi Gong exercises (similar to Tai Chi), as may the practitioner's daily routine. These are designed to put the student or practitioner in touch with their Ki, and in particular in touch with the major energy center located just below the navel in the lower abdomen. Use of this center, the *tanden*, in the middle of the *hara* or abdomen, is an integral part of Shiatsu practice, and therefore hara development is of great importance to both student and practitioner. Indeed, without consciously harnessing the power of hara, it is difficult to give Shiatsu effectively.

The hara and its central focus, the tanden, is in fact the second or sacral chakra, where our physical energy is stored. The Japanese say this is where mind and body come together, and by centering ourselves here we become more balanced and more powerful.

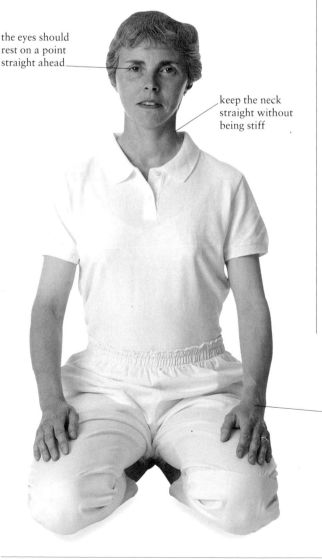

the eyes should rest on a point straight ahead

keep the neck straight without being stiff

rest the hands on the thighs

LEFT *Sitting in Seiza – with the feet under the buttocks and the back straight – is the practitioner's way of centering his or her energy.*

Try these two exercises to see how this can be put into practice:

EXERCISE 1: next time you are running upstairs or to catch a bus, instead of thinking of your aching lungs imagine a ball of light at your hara – you will be able to run faster and longer.

EXERCISE 2: when someone is being angry or upsetting you, instead of reacting emotionally, take your consciousness to hara and breathe deeply – you will now be sufficiently detached to react appropriately.

Relaxed pressure coming from hara allows the Shiatsu giver to be sensitive and yet strong, if necessary; it allows a deeper perception of Ki flow and engages our intuitive capa
which are so important
healing process.

Attention to posture is emphasized in Shiatsu, s comfortable open postu allows the giver's Ki to flow and facilitates the use of hara and the other center that is crucial for compassionate healing, the Heart. Ki awareness, hara development exercises, and meditative practices normally form part of the practitioner's daily routine, along with Shiatsu related stretching or yoga, which all ensure both physical fitness and psychological well-being.

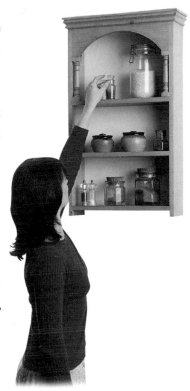

ABOVE *Shiatsu techniques can be used to turn everyday household tasks into energy-releasing stretches.*

Of course practicing Shiatsu itself brings into play the practitioner's own Ki flow. By deep breathing and by applying Ki to the patient, the practitioner's Ki is mobilized, thus stimulating the patient's Ki to flow where it is most needed. When the practitioner's Ki quality is weak or disturbed, this will affect the quality of Shiatsu given; likewise, when the Ki is strong, and the practitioner is "in good form," the ability to stimulate the patient's Ki and promote healing is enhanced.

So we can see that Shiatsu is a two-way process. The practitioner lends skill, experience, and knowledge as a catalyst in the patient's self-healing. The patient lends himself as the medium through which the therapist can practice his or her art. This exchange of energy illustrates one of the prime laws of the universe – that everything is changing and energy is always in a constant state of flow and change.

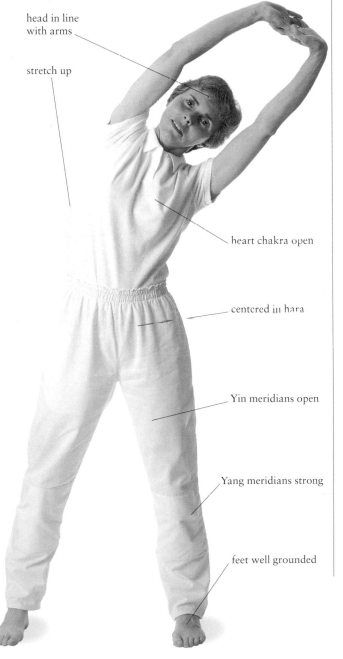

head in line with arms

stretch up

heart chakra open

centered in hara

Yin meridians open

Yang meridians strong

feet well grounded

LEFT *Stretching exercises aid the practitioner in mobilizing his or her own Ki prior to treatment.*

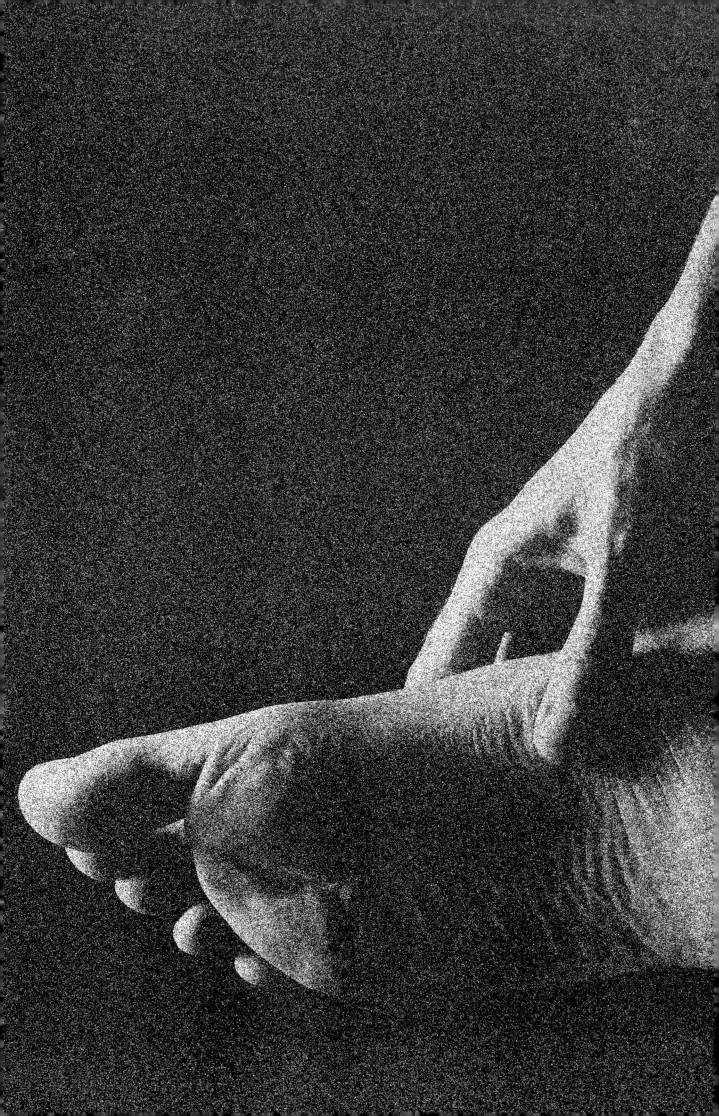

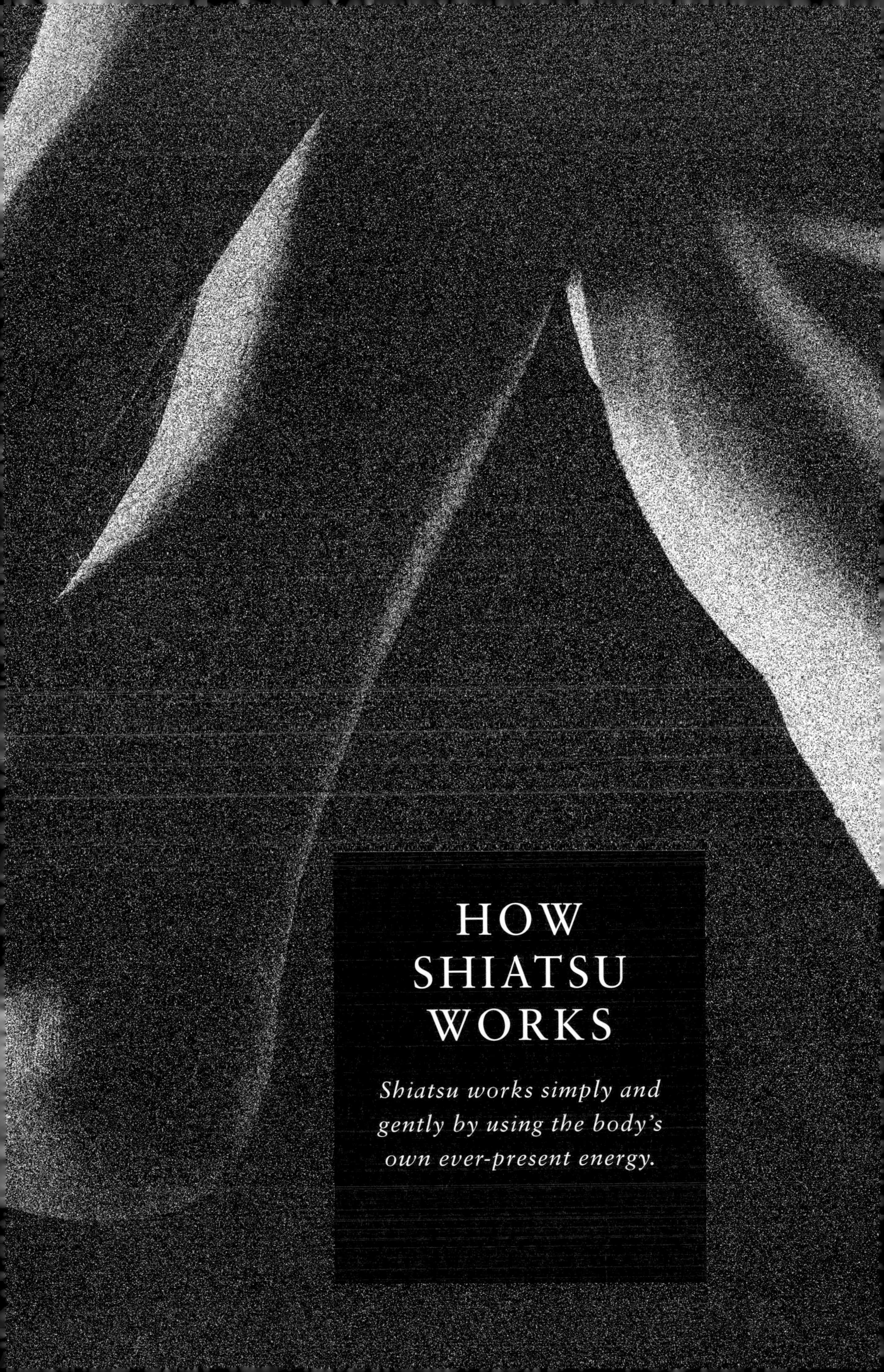

HOW
SHIATSU
WORKS

Shiatsu works simply and
gently by using the body's
own ever-present energy.

▣ Ki Energy

From very ancient times the Chinese have considered the universe to be comprised of energy in various stages of vibration and manifestation. Modern quantum physicists are proving now in their laboratories what the ancient orientals have known for centuries, that Ki energy is found in the tiniest particles that make up the form and substance of our universe. Indeed, those particles, the building blocks of all matter and form, are themselves no more than Ki in vibration. Ki refers to energy in the very widest sense; it is everywhere, in everything, never ending or beginning; it encompasses time, space, matter, form, and movement. Everything is Ki and Ki is everything. Everything that we can conceive of is merely Ki manifesting in a different form, ranging from the most subtle levels: spirit, thought, aura, love, light, air, to the denser and material substances: earth, rock, metal, and animate beings.

For those of us brought up in Western culture, this concept of the whole universe being made essentially of the same "stuff" is an alien and difficult idea. However, if we look at some simple examples, we can easily see how Ki as existence is constantly changing, yet never ceasing to be. A drop of dew that condenses in the cool of night warms up and vaporizes during the day, rising to form a cloud, where it may freeze into a hailstone, fall to earth, and melt back into water… A piece of wood is thrown on a fire, it burns and floats into the air as smoke and ash; the ash settles on the earth, where it forms part of the soil and feeds a seed that becomes a tree, which is

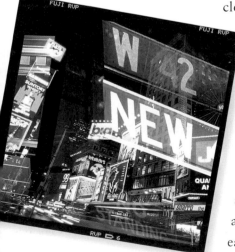

ABOVE *Energy is all around us, but we often overlook our own.*

cut for firewood… These are two very simple examples of how things change in form and substance, yet the energy that constitutes them continues to exist.

A more complex and long-term illustration might be the creation of a human being through the sexual activity of a man and woman. The cluster of cells grows to form a perfect human body, which emerges into the world as a child. Within the maturing person, cells are constantly dying and being renewed so that the full-grown adult is not the same substance in terms of flesh, blood, and bone as the little child, yet he or she is the same person. Eventually the person dies and the body decomposes into the ground, while the spirit returns to what the Chinese would term "the Great Void." (Shiatsu, by the way, does not have any views about the hereafter and is therefore perfectly compatible with any religion or philosophical outlook.)

We can see from these examples that things in existence are in a continual state of transformation; even the processes of life, growth, and death are themselves only changes of form at a very elementary cellular level. What is common to all is Ki. Ki is the energetic substance of all things, it is also the force underlying all change and movement. In short, our entire universe is composed of Ki manifesting in an infinite number of forms and stages of materialization. Ki is "the One" referred to in the quotation by Lao Tzu at the start of this chapter, and it is interesting that most religions have an emphasis on the number one: the acknowledgement of one God, or the attaining of oneness.

THE TRANSFORMATION OF KI ENERGY

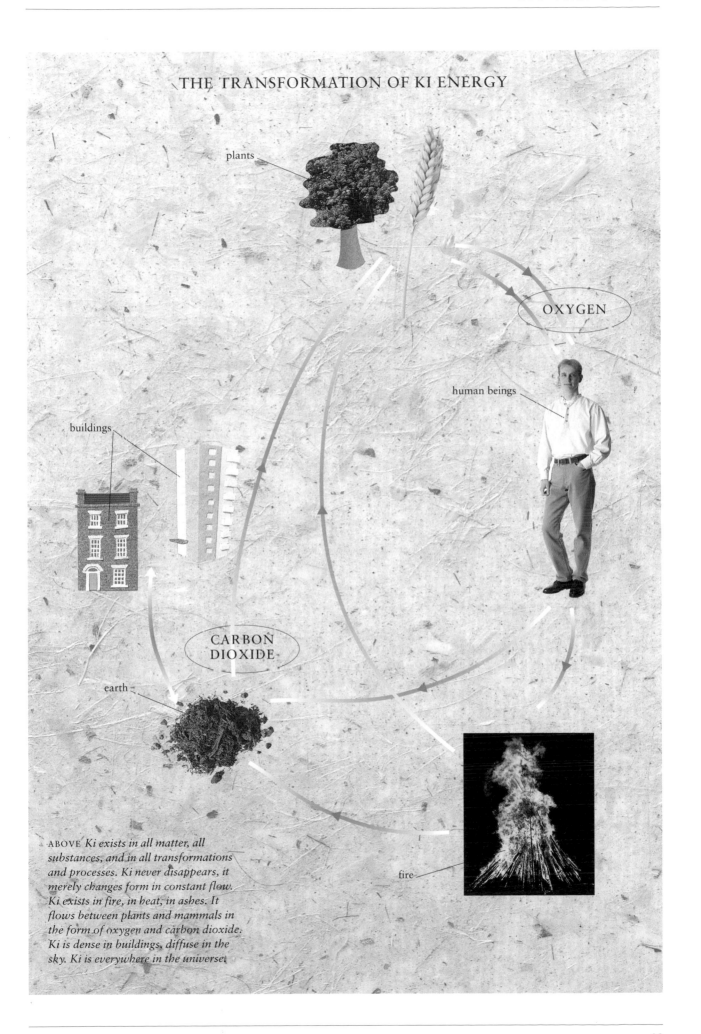

plants

OXYGEN

human beings

buildings

CARBON DIOXIDE

earth

fire

ABOVE *Ki exists in all matter, all substances, and in all transformations and processes. Ki never disappears, it merely changes form in constant flow. Ki exists in fire, in heat, in ashes. It flows between plants and mammals in the form of oxygen and carbon dioxide. Ki is dense in buildings, diffuse in the sky. Ki is everywhere in the universe.*

2 Yin and Yang

"The One begets the Two." Thus the Ki of the universe at the beginning of time differentiated into two forces, Yin and Yang. The quality of Yang was more rarified, immaterial, and more vast, it therefore floated upward to form the Heavens. Yin was more condensed and material, it sank down and created Earth. Thus the ancient Chinese philosophers explained the creation of the world.

The theory of Yin Yang describes how Ki differentiates into different qualities, and how these forces interact. We should note that this is a theory, a human intellectual construction that we can use to describe and make sense of the real world as we experience it. Yin Yang is both a way of summing up the movement of Ki, describing how the universe works, and it is also a way of thinking. It is an all-encompassing theory and at the same time a simple tool which, once learned, can be used to explain any number of phenomena; for example, why some people get on well together and others don't, why certain people tend toward a certain hobby or activity, why you may keep getting the same kind of health problem, how political and economic changes come about, how the moon affects the ocean tides… and so on, the possibilities are endless.

If we look at the symbol for Yin Yang, we can see that it perfectly illustrates the principles that are essential to the theory.

1. The circle symbolizes the wholeness and infinity of Ki, having neither beginning nor ending, and pervading everything.

2. The line dividing the two forces is a curved one, denoting movement and the constant flow of Yin into Yang and vice versa.

3. Within each color is a dot of the opposing one. This shows that there are no absolutes and that everything contains the seeds of its opposite within it. Yin and Yang may be opposites, but they cannot exist without each other: there is no up without down, no hot without cold. Also, each Yin and Yang can be further broken down relative to each other; therefore, within hot we have tepid (more yin), and fiery hot (more yang), within cold moderately cold (more yang) and icy (more yin).

4. The two colors are in equal proportion, making a dynamic balance. When there is more of one aspect, there is less of the other, and at their extremes they transform into each other.

The dynamic of Yin Yang is therefore very flexible. Its qualities are not exclusive, but complementary and relative. Life is not simply black and white, but a scale of colors going from one end of the spectrum to the other and always changing.

The original meaning for Yin and Yang were "the shady side of a hill" and the "sunny side of a hill," respectively. Yin therefore was associated with darkness, coldness, resting, quietness. Yang was the opposite: light, heat, activity, movement. By the further association of Yang with Heaven and Yin with the Earth, a whole series of qualities were assigned to each category.

THE PRINCIPAL QUALITIES

YIN		YANG	
	EARTH		HEAVEN
	DARK		LIGHT
	COLD		HOT
	DAMP		DRY
	MOON		SUN
	WATER		FIRE
	PASSIVE		ACTIVE
	REST		MOVEMENT
	SOFT		HARD
	CONTRACTION		EXPANSION
	SINKING		RISING
	MATERIAL		IMMATERIAL
	FEMALE		MALE

LEFT *The original meaning of Yin and Yang – the shady and sunny sides of a hill – captures their differences and complementary elements.*

Yin Yang Medical Theory

In regard to medicine, Yin Yang is the fundamental principle used to diagnose the individual's state of Ki and to describe the nature and location of illness. Within the body, Yin and Yang qualities can be categorized as follows:

Yin Yang tends to be used as an overall general guide to the state of a person's Ki. We all have a constitutional tendency to be either more Yin or more Yang in nature. If in the shorter term, however, either the Yin or the Yang forces greatly predominate in a person's body or mind, then he or she will have an imbalance, and this will lead to symptoms of one sort of another.

Using Yin Yang theory we can sum up a person's constitution or long-term tendencies, and their condition, or short-term symptoms.

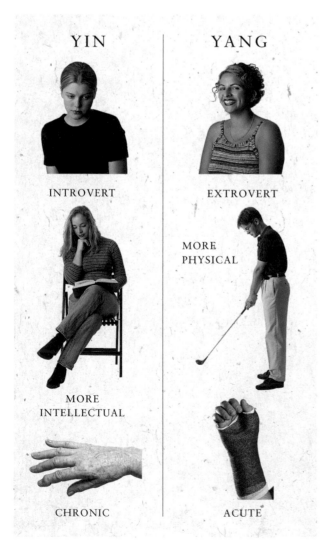

YIN

INTROVERT

MORE
INTELLECTUAL

CHRONIC

YANG

EXTROVERT

MORE
PHYSICAL

ACUTE

YIN YANG SYMPTOM IMBALANCES

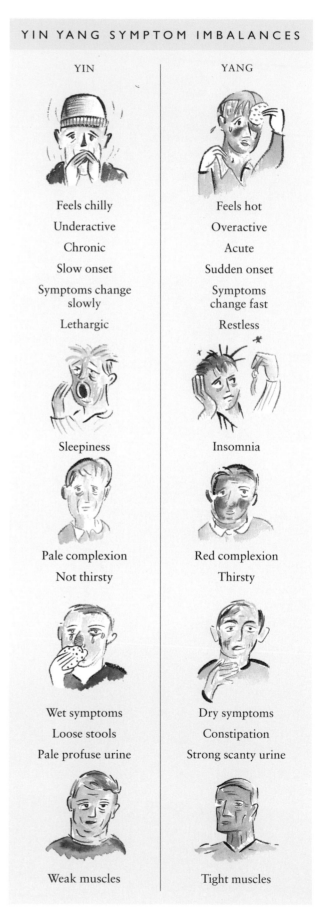

YIN	YANG
Feels chilly	Feels hot
Underactive	Overactive
Chronic	Acute
Slow onset	Sudden onset
Symptoms change slowly	Symptoms change fast
Lethargic	Restless
Sleepiness	Insomnia
Pale complexion	Red complexion
Not thirsty	Thirsty
Wet symptoms	Dry symptoms
Loose stools	Constipation
Pale profuse urine	Strong scanty urine
Weak muscles	Tight muscles

YIN

YANG

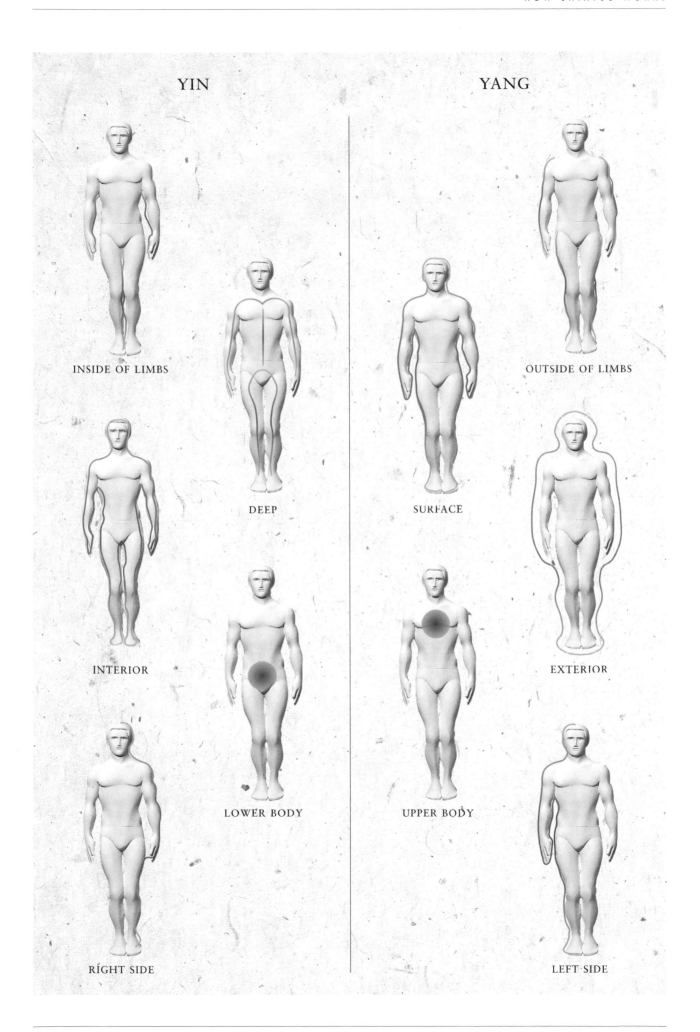

INSIDE OF LIMBS

DEEP

SURFACE

OUTSIDE OF LIMBS

INTERIOR

LOWER BODY

UPPER BODY

EXTERIOR

RIGHT SIDE

LEFT SIDE

3 The Five Elements

The Five Elements represent a further classification of Yin and Yang into different forms of Ki, described by the qualities of Metal, Water, Wood, Fire, and Earth. Although these appear similar to the old alchemical elements known in the West (Earth, Air, Fire, and Water), we should note that the word "element" in English has a somewhat fixed connotation that is not present in the Chinese; hence the theory is often known by the alternative translations of Five Transformations or Five Phases. The Elements themselves are in fact descriptions of Ki in different stages and processes of change. For practitioners of Shiatsu and other forms of oriental medicine, Five Element theory is a very useful model to work with because it is more tangible and therefore easier to grasp than the sometimes nebulous feeling qualities of Yin Yang. Like Yin Yang, the Five Element view of the universe arose from observing the cycles of nature and categorizing the interaction of phenomena.

Five Element theory comprises two aspects; firstly, the grouping together of things or phenomena with a similar energy quality into "correspondences," and secondly, the flow of energy between the Elements in very defined sequences or cycles. Each Element has its own characteristic properties and qualities that we can understand on an intuitive and common-sense level.

◎ WOOD energy, for example, is the rising, expanding, and growing feeling we are aware of in the spring when nature awakens from the long sleep of winter and the great surge of activity and growth that starts the year begins.

◎ FIRE quality is the ultimate Yang of high summer, when nature is at its peak of growth; the trees are in full leaf and flowers bloom.

◎ EARTH is the element of center and balance, where the energy starts to transform into a downward movement; it is associated with late or Indian summer and also with the last few days of each season, when the Ki of the season starts to change into the next.

◎ METAL energy is consolidating and inward-moving, like sap in the fall. It condenses things into their constituent parts and creates the boundaries that define them; like a fall mist lying in a valley, created by the condensation of water but unable to rise up and transform itself by evaporation.

◎ WATER is the ultimate Yin; the quiet, cold, resting time of winter. It has a waiting, still quality that could be described as "stored potential," yet it is always capable of flexibility (think of water filling up any shape of vessel) and has great power (think of the devastation left by floods).

The Five Element correspondences group together phenomena that are seen to have a similar energy quality, like a group of musical instruments all playing the same note.

When applied to the realm of the human body, mind, and spirit Five Elements can be an invaluable tool in pinpointing where and how the body's Ki has become imbalanced.

We shall look at the practical application of the Five Element correspondences a little further on in this chapter (see pp. 60–61) and then again when we look at some case histories, as part of the Basic Sequence (see p. 106).

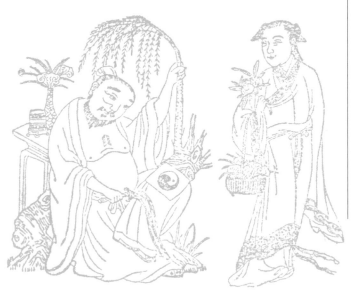

LEFT *This Chinese drawing shows the Yang (male) and Yin (female) types.*

Table of General Correspondences

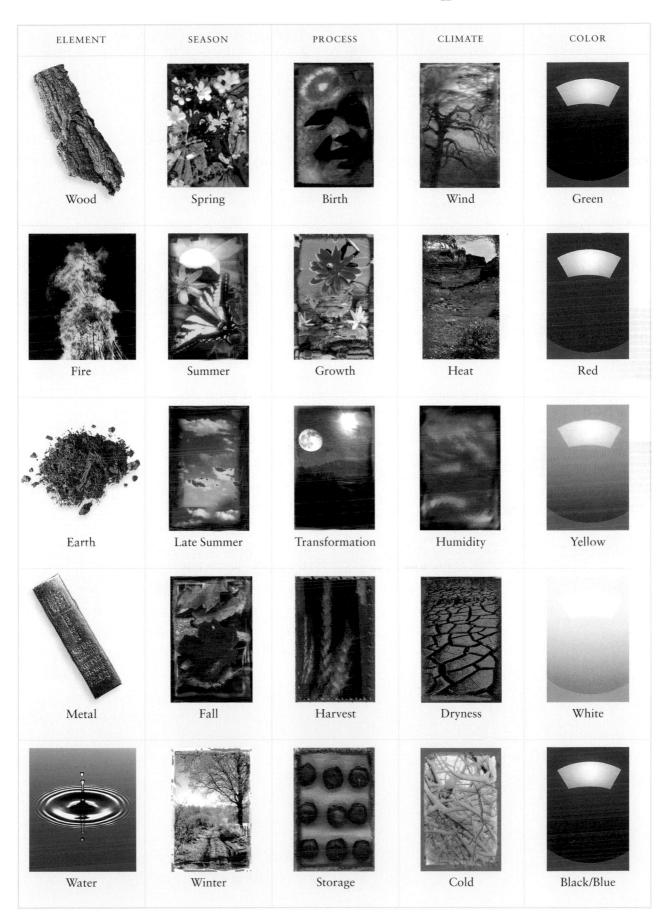

ELEMENT	SEASON	PROCESS	CLIMATE	COLOR
Wood	Spring	Birth	Wind	Green
Fire	Summer	Growth	Heat	Red
Earth	Late Summer	Transformation	Humidity	Yellow
Metal	Fall	Harvest	Dryness	White
Water	Winter	Storage	Cold	Black/Blue

Table of Human Correspondences

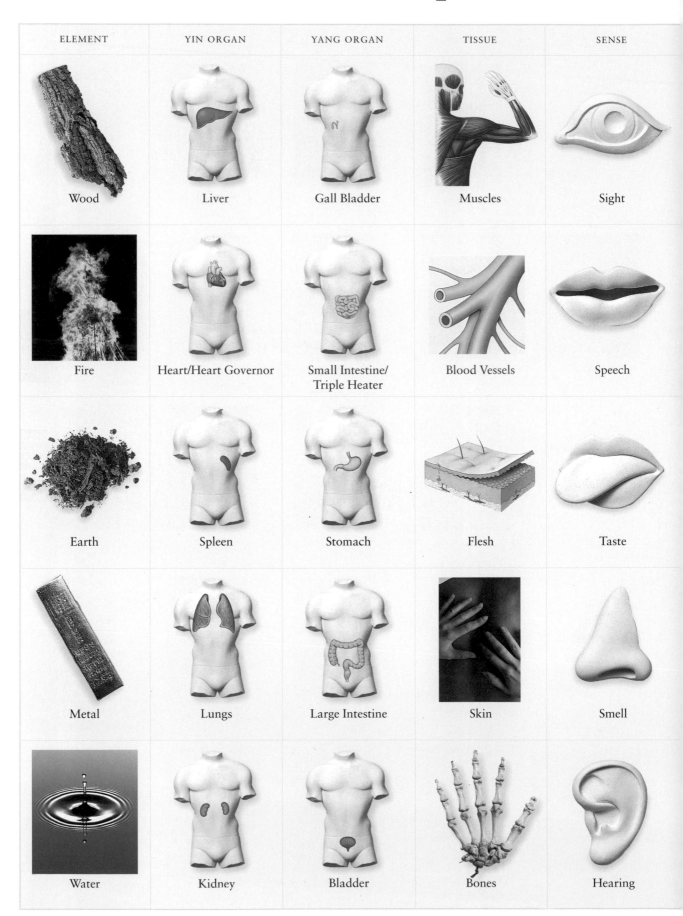

ELEMENT	YIN ORGAN	YANG ORGAN	TISSUE	SENSE
Wood	Liver	Gall Bladder	Muscles	Sight
Fire	Heart/Heart Governor	Small Intestine/ Triple Heater	Blood Vessels	Speech
Earth	Spleen	Stomach	Flesh	Taste
Metal	Lungs	Large Intestine	Skin	Smell
Water	Kidney	Bladder	Bones	Hearing

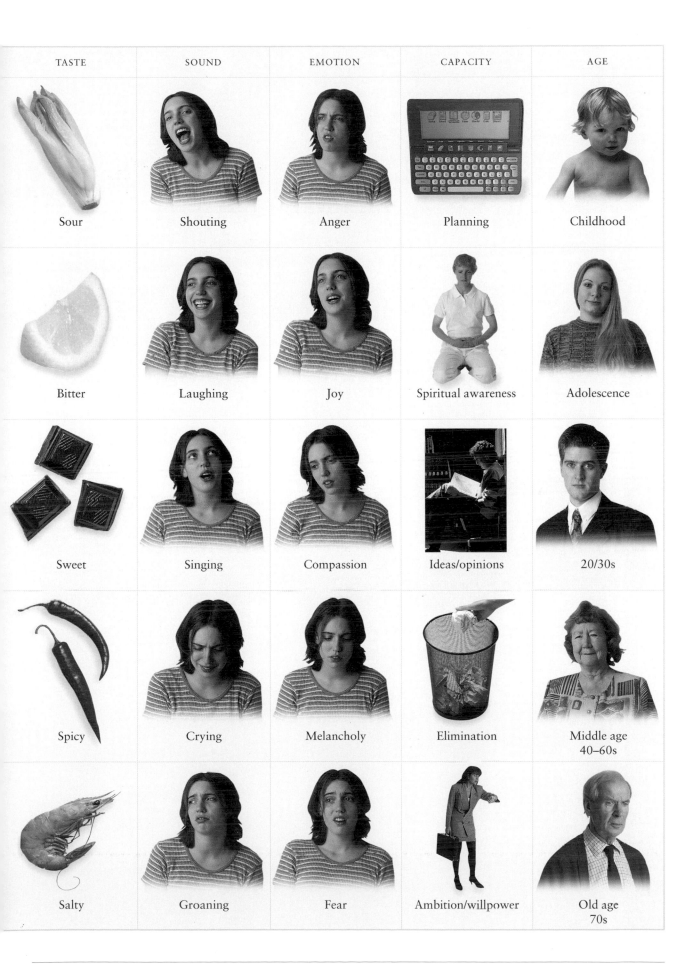

TASTE	SOUND	EMOTION	CAPACITY	AGE
Sour	Shouting	Anger	Planning	Childhood
Bitter	Laughing	Joy	Spiritual awareness	Adolescence
Sweet	Singing	Compassion	Ideas/opinions	20/30s
Spicy	Crying	Melancholy	Elimination	Middle age 40–60s
Salty	Groaning	Fear	Ambition/willpower	Old age 70s

Ki's Cyclical Flow

The second important aspect of Five Element theory is its very specific description of the way energy flows around a Yin Yang circle in nature. Ki moves in a cyclical fashion, with each Element generating or flowing into the next one in what is known as the Creative (Shen) cycle. Wood (growing Yang) therefore creates or generates Fire (extreme Yang), which settles down into Earth (Yang turning toward Yin), Earth condenses down into Metal (solid Yin), which melts into Water (fluid Yin), Water flows into Wood, and so the cycle goes on.

The cycle of the seasons is a good example of the Creative cycle. In the spring (Wood energy time), there is tremendous energetic activity in growing plants and trees bursting into leaf; this culminates in the high activity of summer (Fire), with fruit and flowers at their peak. Inevitably, the surge of activity tires into late Indian summer (Earth time) when the fruit ripens, then the Ki of the earth mellows into the harvest time of fall (Metal) when the leaves fall from the trees. This consolidating phase transforms to the cold of winter (Water), when life seems to stop and regroup, ready to begin the whole process again.

The pattern of our activity through life is another example of this natural cycle, with childhood growth representing Wood, Fire the emotional turbulence of adolescence, Earth the maturity of our reproductive years, Metal the consolidation of our achievements, and the quiet time of Water the precursor to our long sleep after death.

In models or diagrams of the creative cycle, each of the Elements is given equal space. In practice, however, one phase may pass quite slowly while another might last only minutes. Imagine, for example, being nearly knocked off your bicycle on a busy road. Momentary fright (Water) is almost immediately replaced by anger (Wood), lasting some considerable time. Later, relief or joy (Fire) gives way to a few moments of self-pity (Earth) that you can't afford a car, but you find a new sense of positivity (Metal) as you continue pedaling, knowing you're taking good exercise.

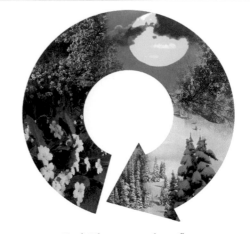

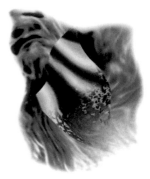

Each Element or phase flows naturally into the next.

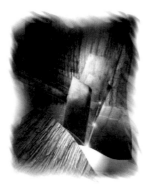

Wood: *The outward surge of Wood Ki expands into the all-encompassing warmth of Fire.*

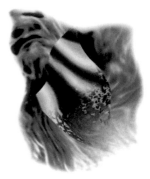

Fire: *After the ultimate expansion of Fire, Ki transforms to the inward gathering of Earth.*

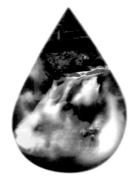

Water: *The ultimate flexibility of liquid Ki nourishes the upward growth of Wood.*

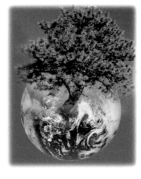

Earth: *The centering quality of Earth energy feeds the consolidating movement of Metal.*

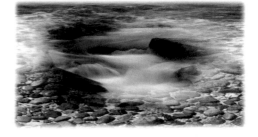

Metal: *The solidity and extreme material condensation of Metal relaxes into the fluidity of water.*

THE CREATIVE AND CONTROL CYCLES

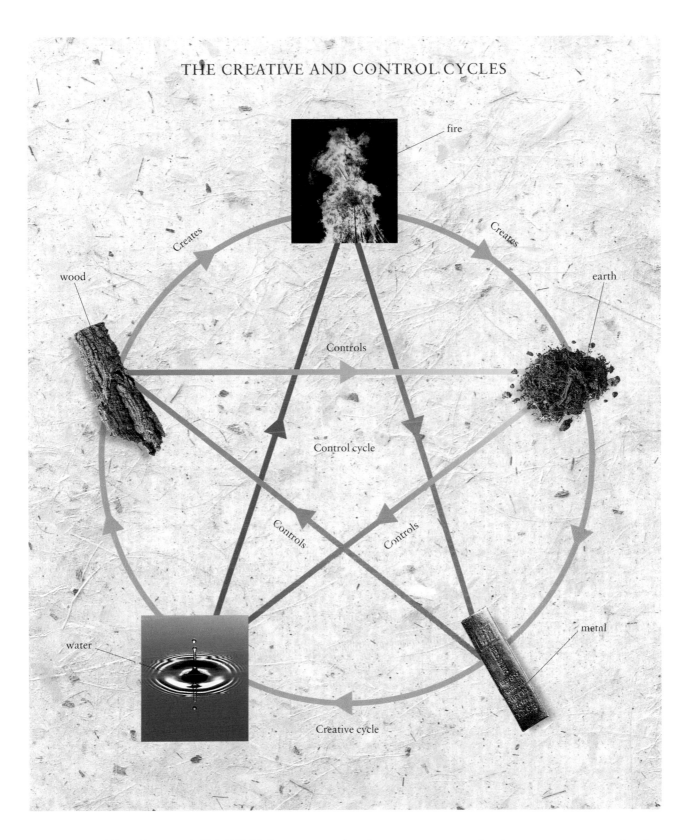

fire

wood

earth

Creates

Creates

Controls

Control cycle

Controls

Controls

water

metal

Creative cycle

THE LIMITING EFFECT OF KO

This creative mechanism would continue to increase infinitely were it not for another energetic cycle holding the creative forces in check and limiting their effect. This is the Control (Ko) cycle, symbolically drawn as a five-pointed star within the circle of the Creative cycle. Governed by this process the Elements restrain each other again in a natural order. Here Fire modifies the structure of Metal by melting it; Metal contains the exuberance of Wood by cutting it or boxing it in; Wood (creative growing energy) lightens the stable gravity of Earth; Earth limits the flow of Water by damming it up; and Water puts out Fire.

Five Element Theory as a Life-guide

Like all theories, these two cycles are merely descriptions of observed reality, just as a map is not the actual countryside on which you walk. Using theory as a guide can help to make sense of the terrain, but we should not confuse the theory (what ought to happen) with reality (what does happen). The basic lie of the land may not change, but landmarks such as trees or hedges may be cut down, or footpaths may become blocked or overgrown, so that the actual place may not correspond exactly with the map. We all contain and express each of the Elements in different measure in our personal makeup and we move through the cycles of the Elements at different rates, depending on our energetic structure. So a Fire-type person may be comfortable living life in the high activity of emotional turmoil, just as Fire-type people want summer to go on forever. Whereas an Earth-type person like me dislikes summer with its heat and unstructured "busy-ness," and therefore welcomes the stability of the new school term, beginning in the Earth time of late summer.

Sometimes we go through an Element phase on the Creative cycle so fast that we barely even notice moving through it. However, at other times, we may get stuck in a phase and require the modifying forces of the Control cycle to limit the increasing tendency of the Creative cycle; for example, the longterm depressive grief that is experienced after a bereavement – Metal – may be lightened by compassionate spiritual comfort – Fire.

The Creative and Control cycles are an expression of the natural balances of energy in the universe, but when Ki goes out of balance, these cycles may be distorted. In particular, the Control cycle may over-control the Element it is supposed to limit, so that it can no longer function normally, or, if the control is excessive, the controlled Element may rebel and "insult" its controller. For instance, Fire is normally put out by Water, but if out of control it well may evaporate Water. This will be covered further in the Diagnosis section.

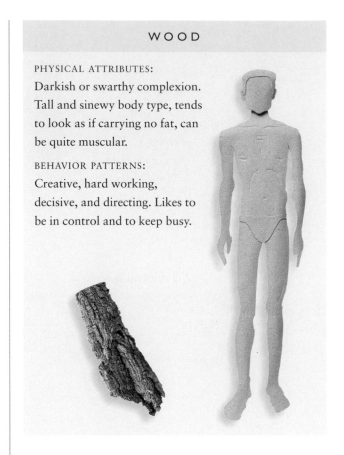

WOOD

PHYSICAL ATTRIBUTES:
Darkish or swarthy complexion. Tall and sinewy body type, tends to look as if carrying no fat, can be quite muscular.

BEHAVIOR PATTERNS:
Creative, hard working, decisive, and directing. Likes to be in control and to keep busy.

FIVE ELEMENT TYPES

Human beings contain and express the energy of all five Elements within their physical and psycho-emotional makeup. A person's individuality is created by the particular balance and mixture of Elemental energy manifested both in the long term (in a person's constitution inherited from his or her parents), in the short term (a person's current condition). Everyone has a tendency to favor one Element or a certain combination of Elements in their health patterns and way of dealing with life.

In traditional theory there are Element "types" which encapsulate the characteristics of each Element in terms of physical appearance and behavior patterns. A knowledge of these types can help people to recognize themselves and others. In the descriptions given here the typical balanced attributes of the Elements are given: imbalances can be deduced from the section on Meridians and their related associations and imbalances (see pp. 70–73).

FIRE

PHYSICAL ATTRIBUTES:
Red complexion. Head often smallish and pointed, or may have a pointed chin. Hair is often curly, in men a tendency to baldness. Hands and feet tend to be small and graceful. Walks quickly.

BEHAVIOR PATTERNS:
Emotional, communicative, and articulate. Tends to be very sociable, loving, and can be quite spiritual in outlook.

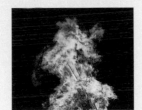

METAL

PHYSICAL ATTRIBUTES:
Pale complexion with smooth and clear skin. Angular, well-defined features. Broad chest and shoulders. Abundant body hair. Tends to walk slowly.

BEHAVIOR PATTERNS:
Well-organized, neat, methodical, and meticulous. Tends to be very self-contained and does not express emotion much.

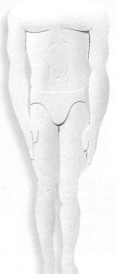

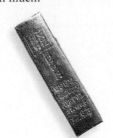

EARTH

PHYSICAL ATTRIBUTES:
Brownish or sallow complexion with a large head. Tends to be pear shaped, carrying weight in the hips. Muscular or fat with heavy legs. Does not lift feet high when walking.

BEHAVIOR PATTERNS:
Sympathetic, considerate, and supportive. Tends to be an "Earth Mother" type, with focus on caring for others.

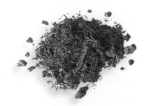

WATER

PHYSICAL ATTRIBUTES:
High forehead and abundant head hair. Long, strong bone structure with spine proportionately longer than normal. Fluid movement.

BEHAVIOR PATTERNS:
Flexible, well-motivated, ambitious. Can also tend to be lazy and "go with the flow" too much.

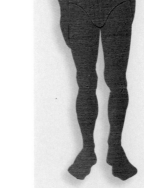

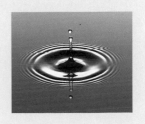

4 How Ki Works in the Body

When we apply the generalized theories of Yin Yang and the Five Elements to the body, they provide us with a very apt description of the ways in which Ki flows and balances. Good health requires a free and harmonious flow of Ki throughout all parts of the body, like a network of rivers and streams flowing steadily through the countryside. And because the mind, emotions, and spirit are merely a less dense aspect of the individual's material bodily Ki, when Ki is flowing smoothly in the body it is also balanced in mind and spirit. This is the essence of the holistic approach of oriental medicine and Shiatsu in particular: that we can feel the imbalance of Ki by touching the body, no matter at which level (physical, emotional, spiritual) the imbalance is occurring, and that by the use of technique – pressure, rubbing, and stretching – we can realign the imbalanced Ki.

Ki comes to us from three basic sources. Original Ki comes from our parents; we could say it is our genetic inheritance and our basic constitution. Grain Ki is the Ki we ingest from our food. Air Ki is derived through breathing. These three together compromise our overall Ki quality.

Chinese acupuncture theory has a whole complex classification of different manifestations of Ki in the body-mind, which practitioners of Shiatsu are aware of, but it is unnecessary for us to go into them here. The only two aspects of Ki that will be useful for us to note are Jing and Shen. These are Chinese terms, and in Shiatsu we tend to use these rather than their Japanese equivalent. Jing is the essential energy that governs the long-term processes of growth, maturation, and death. It is responsible for our ability to have children and the pace at which we age. Jing resides in the kidneys. Shen is translated as either the "spirit" or the "mind" but in reality encompasses both of these facets of ourselves. It is to do with our emotions and also the human awareness and consciousness that make up our individual personality. The Shen is said to reside in the heart.

protective Ki
on skin surface

KI HAS FIVE BASIC FUNCTIONS IN THE BODY

Movement: in other words, any form of activity, whether physical or mental, voluntary or involuntary.

Protection: it protects the body from outside influences such as cold, wind, infections, and so on.

Warmth: Ki keeps all parts of the body warm, regulating overall temperature and also peripheral circulation.

Transformation: it is Ki that changes food into the various building blocks we need for good health.

Retention: keeping the organs in their proper places, preventing prolapse, holding blood in the blood vessels, and so on.

CAUSES OF IMBALANCE

What is it that causes Ki to become imbalanced or disturbed in the body-mind? In reality there is never one cause, but a network of factors that may combine to manifest in a particular pattern of imbalance. Oriental medicine basically classifies the sources of imbalance into internal or emotional factors, external or climatic factors, and lifestyle or miscellaneous factors.

The seven principal emotions are *joy, sadness, fear, fright, worry, overthinking,* and *anger.* Each is associated with a particular meridian; for example, joy affects the heart, anger affects the liver, fear affects the kidneys, and so on. These associations are detailed in the section on meridian imbalance further on in this chapter (see pp. 70–73).

movement
creates warmth

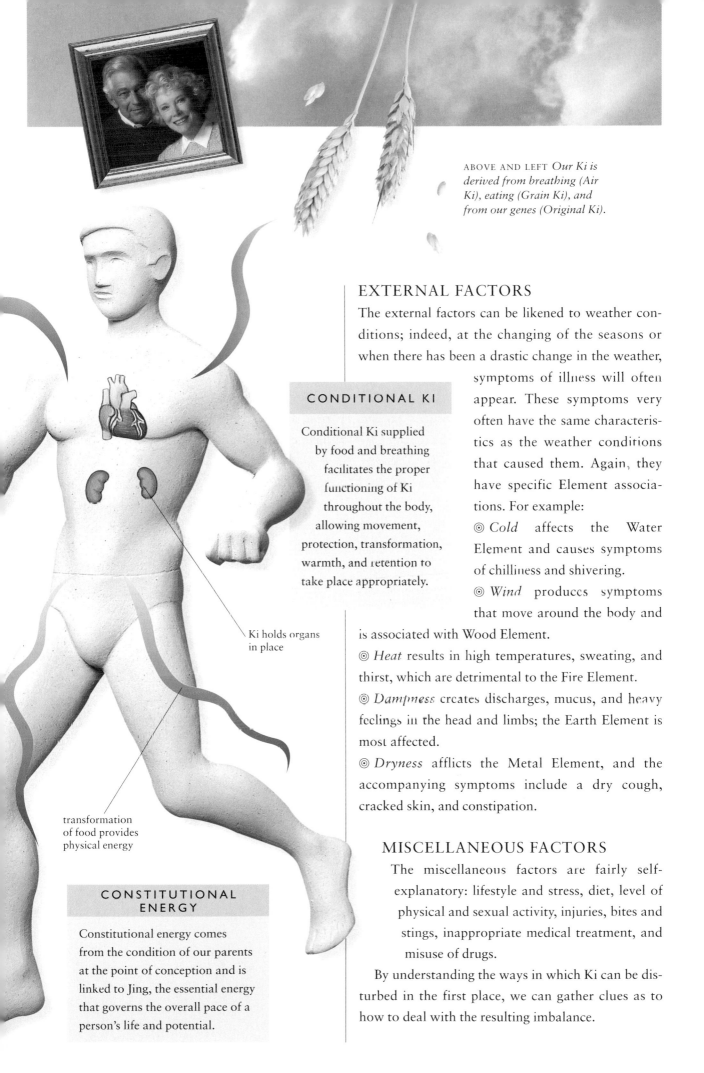

ABOVE AND LEFT *Our Ki is
derived from breathing (Air
Ki), eating (Grain Ki), and
from our genes (Original Ki).*

Ki holds organs
in place

transformation
of food provides
physical energy

CONDITIONAL KI

Conditional Ki supplied
by food and breathing
facilitates the proper
functioning of Ki
throughout the body,
allowing movement,
protection, transformation,
warmth, and retention to
take place appropriately.

CONSTITUTIONAL
ENERGY

Constitutional energy comes
from the condition of our parents
at the point of conception and is
linked to Jing, the essential energy
that governs the overall pace of a
person's life and potential.

EXTERNAL FACTORS

The external factors can be likened to weather conditions; indeed, at the changing of the seasons or
when there has been a drastic change in the weather,
symptoms of illness will often
appear. These symptoms very
often have the same characteristics as the weather conditions
that caused them. Again, they
have specific Element associations. For example:

◎ *Cold* affects the Water
Element and causes symptoms
of chilliness and shivering.

◎ *Wind* produces symptoms
that move around the body and
is associated with Wood Element.

◎ *Heat* results in high temperatures, sweating, and
thirst, which are detrimental to the Fire Element.

◎ *Dampness* creates discharges, mucus, and heavy
feelings in the head and limbs; the Earth Element is
most affected.

◎ *Dryness* afflicts the Metal Element, and the
accompanying symptoms include a dry cough,
cracked skin, and constipation.

MISCELLANEOUS FACTORS

The miscellaneous factors are fairly self-
explanatory: lifestyle and stress, diet, level of
physical and sexual activity, injuries, bites and
stings, inappropriate medical treatment, and
misuse of drugs.

By understanding the ways in which Ki can be disturbed in the first place, we can gather clues as to
how to deal with the resulting imbalance.

The Meridians

Ki moves throughout the whole body, but in certain defined pathways it flows in a more concentrated manner. These pathways are known as the meridians. The meridians form a continuous circuit of lines that allows the flow of different aspects of Ki all over the body. Each meridian is named after a physical organ, for example the Heart meridian, Lung meridian, and Bladder meridian. However, the meridian does not just relate to the physical organ, but encompasses a whole constellation of meanings based around a particular function. Indeed, the easiest way to define a meridian is in terms of function. Rather than think of the meridian as a pathway attached to an organ, we should look on the meridian as a concentration of a particular functional energetic quality of the body. Where it reaches its most intense point, there it creates a physical organ to carry out that function. Knowledge of where the meridians run has been developed through centuries of observation and clinical experience, and nowadays their energy can be measured scientifically with electronic instruments. Shiatsu practitioners learn, over time, to feel the meridians through increased sensitivity of touch.

There are 12 meridians that run on both sides of the body and two central channels; (see pp. 66–7). The meridians are classified according to their function. If you imagine someone standing with arms stretched up to the sky, the Yang meridians run from the "Great Yang" of Heaven down the back and outsides of the body, whereas the Yin meridians run from the "Great Yin," the Earth, up the front and insides of the limbs. Each Element has a particular energetic quality that governs a particular function. This is carried out by a pair of meridians that are in effect the Yin and Yang aspects of the same function or Ki quality, like two sides of the same coin. The following table shows the functions of the meridians using Zen Shiatsu theory (which I use in my practice). The Five Element human correspondences table shows some of the connections (see pp. 56–7).

The order in which the meridians are listed here is different from the order of the Five Elements flow using the Creative cycle. This is because in meridian theory, Ki runs from one meridian to the next in a continuous loop, so the Lung meridian ends close to where Large Intestine starts; where Large Intestine finishes the Stomach begins, and so on.

FUNCTIONS OF THE MERIDIANS			
ELEMENT	MERIDIAN	ASPECT	FUNCTION
Metal	Lung Large Intestine	Yin Yang	Intake of Ki (air) and Vitality Elimination
Earth	Stomach Spleen/Pancreas	Yang Yin	Intake of nourishment Digestion and Transformation
Fire (primary)	Heart Small Intestine	Yin Yang	Emotional/Spiritual Center Assimilation
Water	Bladder Kidneys	Yang Yin	Purification Impetus
Fire (secondary)	Heart Governor Triple Heater	Yin Yang	Circulation Protection
Wood	Gall bladder Liver	Yang Yin	Decision-making and Distribution Control and planning, Detoxification

The Chinese Clock Cycle

Each meridian is also associated with a particular two hour period during the day, when Ki, which circulates continuously, reaches a peak for that channel and its organ. This can be a useful tool in diagnosis to help pinpoint someone's strengths and weaknesses, and in treatment can be used to choose the most effective time to work on a particular meridian. For instance, in my "night owl" phases I can quite happily work until 3 a.m. because my Gall Bladder and Liver energy are fairly strong and keep me going through the night. However, I find I have slumps of energy between 9–11 a.m. and 1 3 p.m., as SP and SI respectively are somewhat low. A good time for me to receive Shiatsu treatment would therefore be at 9–11 a.m. when Spleen energy could be most appropriately tonified, or between 1–3 p.m., when Small Intestine would be effectively tonified, and Liver (at the opposite side of the cycle, 1–3 a.m.) would more easily be sedated.

THE MERIDIAN CYCLE

According to Chinese Clock theory, Ki flows at its maximum in each of the meridians at the following times of day:

3 a.m. – 5 a.m.	Lungs (LU)
5 a.m. – 7 a.m.	Large Intestine (LI)
7 a.m. – 9 a.m.	Stomach (ST)
9 a.m. – 11 a.m.	Spleen/Pancreas (SP)
11 a.m. – 1 p.m.	Heart (HT)
1 p.m. – 3 p.m.	Small Intestine (SI)
3 p.m. – 5 p.m.	Bladder (BL)
5 p.m. – 7 p.m.	Kidneys (KD)
7 p.m. – 9 p.m.	Heart Governor (HG)
9 p.m. – 11 p.m.	Triple Heater (TH)
11 p.m. – 1 a.m.	Gall Bladder (GB)
1 a.m. – 3 a.m.	Liver (LIV)

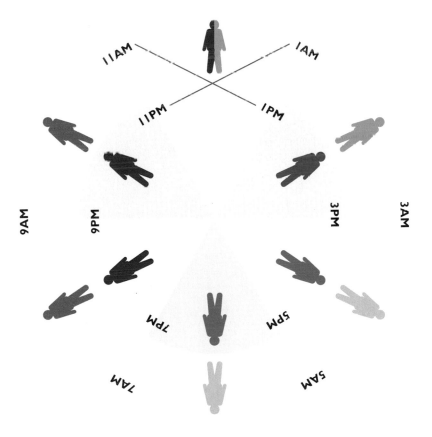

ABOVE *Each meridian is associated with a two-hour period when its energy is at a peak.*

The Meridians

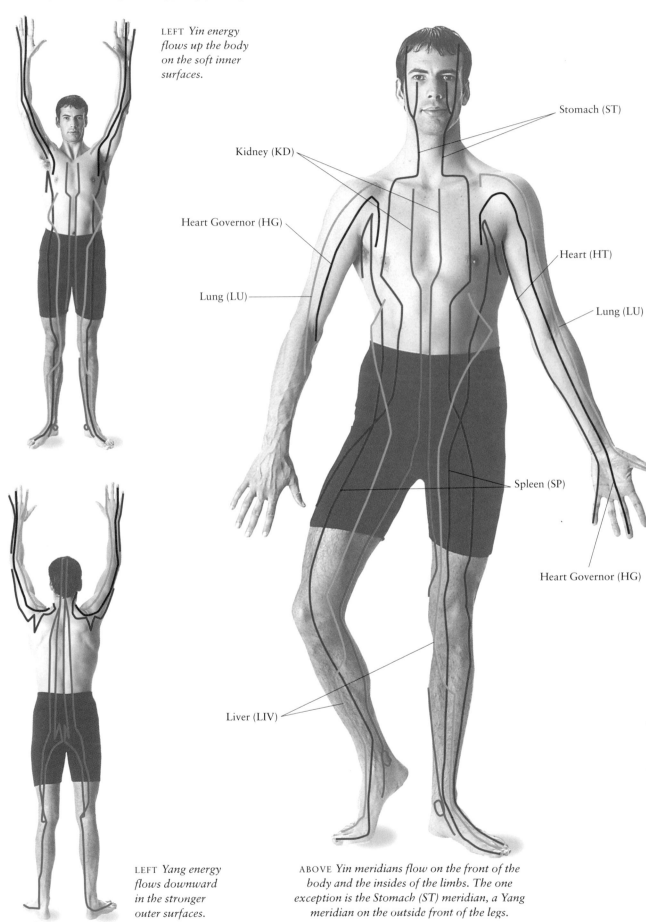

LEFT *Yin energy flows up the body on the soft inner surfaces.*

Stomach (ST)

Kidney (KD)

Heart Governor (HG)

Lung (LU)

Heart (HT)

Lung (LU)

Spleen (SP)

Heart Governor (HG)

Liver (LIV)

LEFT *Yang energy flows downward in the stronger outer surfaces.*

ABOVE *Yin meridians flow on the front of the body and the insides of the limbs. The one exception is the Stomach (ST) meridian, a Yang meridian on the outside front of the legs.*

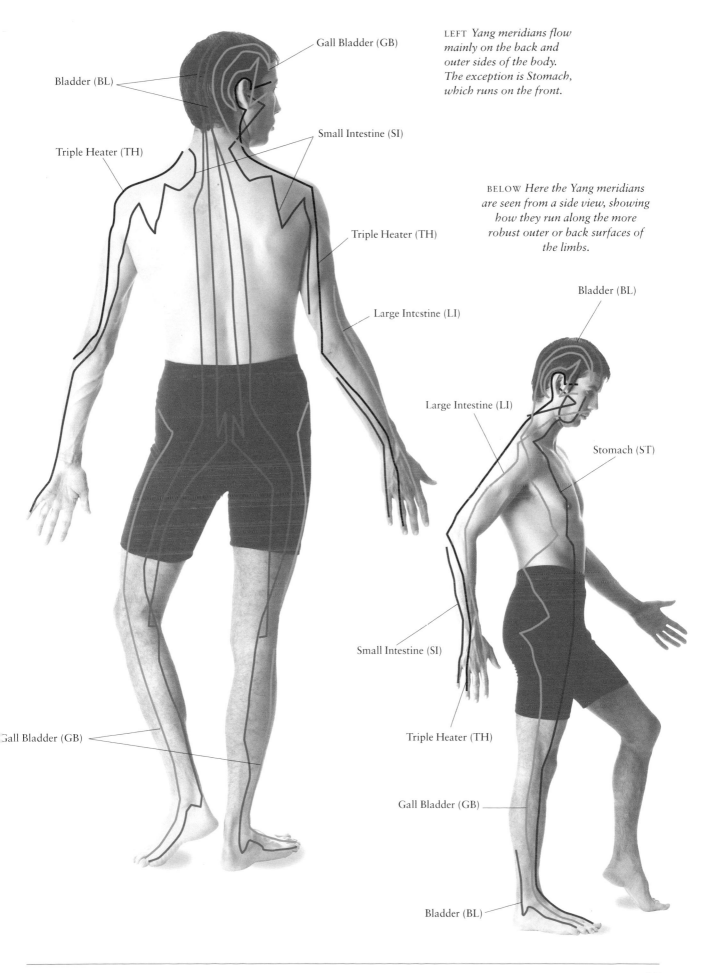

Gall Bladder (GB)

Bladder (BL)

Triple Heater (TH)

Small Intestine (SI)

LEFT Yang meridians flow mainly on the back and outer sides of the body. The exception is Stomach, which runs on the front.

Triple Heater (TH)

BELOW Here the Yang meridians are seen from a side view, showing how they run along the more robust outer or back surfaces of the limbs.

Large Intestine (LI)

Bladder (BL)

Large Intestine (LI)

Stomach (ST)

Small Intestine (SI)

Gall Bladder (GB)

Triple Heater (TH)

Gall Bladder (GB)

Bladder (BL)

Heart Governor and Triple Heater

Before we look at the specific symptoms that may be found as a result of imbalance in any of the meridians, we should explain the nature and function of those two meridians that are not called after any of the physical organs: the Heart Governor and the Triple Heater.

THE HEART GOVERNOR

The Heart Governor is closely related to the heart in its function. Sometimes known as the pericardium (the membranous sheath surrounding the heart) or Heart Protector, like the Heart meridian it governs blood and the circulatory system. However, the Heart Governor has a further protective function that is crucial to its relationship with the heart. The ancient Chinese medical manual known as *The Yellow*

Emperor's Classic of Internal Medicine uses the analogy of the internal organs and meridians being similar to officials within a government in their functions. The heart is likened to the King or Emperor, whose purpose is to safeguard the spiritual and mental stability of his subjects. The heart therefore houses the *Shen* or spiritual and mental faculties. The Heart Governor or Protector is the ambassador who ensures joy and happiness by protecting the King from external harm.

Zen Shiatsu theory equates the Heart Governor slightly more with the physical heart and the circulatory aspects of the cardiac system, whereas the Heart meridian is seen to deal more with the emotional and compassionate, feeling side of ourselves, governing emotional stability and reactions.

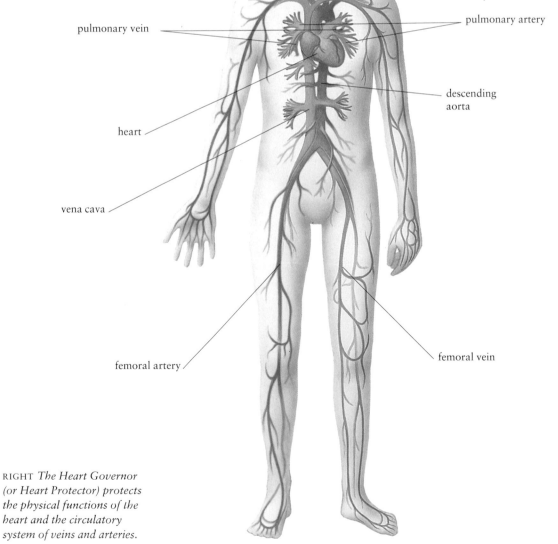

pulmonary vein

pulmonary artery

descending aorta

heart

vena cava

femoral artery

femoral vein

RIGHT *The Heart Governor (or Heart Protector) protects the physical functions of the heart and the circulatory system of veins and arteries.*

THE TRIPLE HEATER

The Triple Heater (Triple Warmer or Triple Burner) has been the subject for much scholarly debate ever since the Chinese started writing about the medical dimensions of Ki. "Triple Heater" is a rather unimaginative translation of "three burning spaces," which refers to the three central chakras: the heart, the solar plexus, and the hara.

Although designated under the Five Elements system as "secondary Fire," the Triple Heater has in fact a close relationship with Water and fluids in the body. *The Yellow Emperor's Classic of Internal Medicine* states: "The Triple Heater is the official in charge of irrigation and it controls the water passages." The same text likens the Upper Heater (governing the heart, lungs, and chest) to a "mist" whose function is to vaporize fluids in the upper body. The Middle Heater is a "foam" and is in charge of transporting nourishment to all parts of the body from the stomach and spleen or pancreas. The Lower Heater (related to the large and small intestines, kidneys, bladder, and liver) is a "swamp" dealing with the transformation, transportation, and excretion of fluids and waste material.

In addition, the Triple Heater acts as the body's thermostat, responsible for our overall temperature, producing and regulating heat throughout the body. Finally, it has a protective function in that many of the points on the TH meridian can be used to defend the body from external factors mentioned in the section on "causes of imbalance," such as Cold, Wind, or Heat.

Masunaga's Zen Shiatsu theory takes all these ideas from traditional Chinese medicine and expands them into modern terms by saying that the Triple Heater also encompasses the functioning of the immune and lymphatic systems, thereby being our body's primary source of protection.

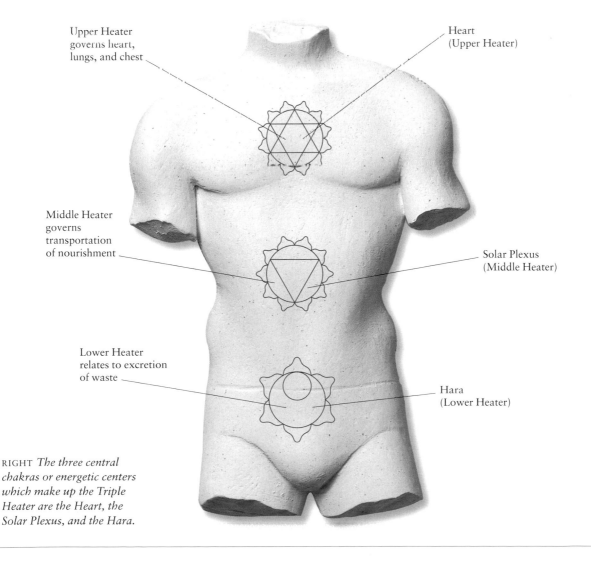

Upper Heater governs heart, lungs, and chest

Heart (Upper Heater)

Middle Heater governs transportation of nourishment

Solar Plexus (Middle Heater)

Lower Heater relates to excretion of waste

Hara (Lower Heater)

RIGHT *The three central chakras or energetic centers which make up the Triple Heater are the Heart, the Solar Plexus, and the Hara.*

Meridian Associations and Imbalances

Let us now look at the detailed function of each meridian, its physical and psychological associations, and the sort of symptoms or conditions that would occur if it were out of balance. As I have said earlier, Shiatsu has several different theoretical approaches. The theory I am presenting here is the particular blend of Zen Shiatsu and Traditional Chinese Medicine that I use in my own practice. I find that in using theory I concentrate on the commonsense and practical applications rather than the esoteric or strictly classical. Therefore, some of the categories below might, on the one hand, not be familiar to a Chinese acupuncturist, and on the other, they might feel I have left out some functions. However, I find that Zen Shiatsu, with its tendency to refine ancient oriental theory and explain it in more modern physiological terms, makes a very satisfactory system to work with. Certainly it seems to

make sense to my patients when I use it to explain their conditions. Again, you may find it useful to refer back to the Five Element human correspondences table (pp. 56–7).

In the tables below, certain very common symptoms of imbalance, like headache, back pain, and anxiety, have not been included. This is because such symptoms may occur in any of the meridians depending on cause and location. Therefore, we would classify, for example, right-sided severe headache as being most likely to be caused by a Gall Bladder imbalance and would treat it quite differently from a fuzzy, "not quite here" frontal headache that might originate in a Spleen or Stomach imbalance. The same can be said for back pain and anxiety: identifying the site of the disturbance would give a guideline as to which meridian is out of balance.

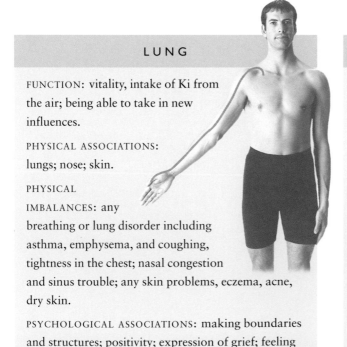

LUNG

FUNCTION: vitality, intake of Ki from the air; being able to take in new influences.

PHYSICAL ASSOCIATIONS: lungs; nose; skin.

PHYSICAL IMBALANCES: any breathing or lung disorder including asthma, emphysema, and coughing, tightness in the chest; nasal congestion and sinus trouble; any skin problems, eczema, acne, dry skin.

PSYCHOLOGICAL ASSOCIATIONS: making boundaries and structures; positivity; expression of grief; feeling of self-worth; self as an individual.

PSYCHOLOGICAL IMBALANCES: isolation and withdrawing; depression, melancholy; negativity, lack of self-worth.

LARGE INTESTINE

FUNCTION: vitality; elimination and excretion.

PHYSICAL ASSOCIATIONS: bowels; skin; nose; sinuses.

PHYSICAL IMBALANCES: any problem relating to the large intestine, including constipation, diarrhea, irritable bowel syndrome, diverticulitis; skin problems; excessive secretion of mucus and catarrh.

PSYCHOLOGICAL ASSOCIATIONS: being able to "let go"; boundaries between self and the outside.

PSYCHOLOGICAL IMBALANCES: inability to "let go," too much "holding on" (physically and mentally); isolation; rigidity or negativity in thinking and outlook.

STOMACH

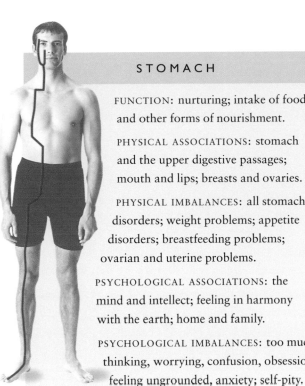

FUNCTION: nurturing; intake of food and other forms of nourishment.

PHYSICAL ASSOCIATIONS: stomach and the upper digestive passages; mouth and lips; breasts and ovaries.

PHYSICAL IMBALANCES: all stomach disorders; weight problems; appetite disorders; breastfeeding problems; ovarian and uterine problems.

PSYCHOLOGICAL ASSOCIATIONS: the mind and intellect; feeling in harmony with the earth; home and family.

PSYCHOLOGICAL IMBALANCES: too much thinking, worrying, confusion, obsession; feeling ungrounded, anxiety; self-pity.

SPLEEN/PANCREAS

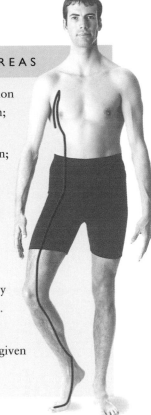

FUNCTION: nurturing; transportation and transformation of Ki; digestion; reproductive cycles.

PHYSICAL ASSOCIATIONS: digestion; appetite; flesh and fat; menstrual cycle; controlling blood.

PHYSICAL IMBALANCES: digestive problems involving insufficient or excessive secretion of digestive enzymes; overeating or lack of appetite; irregular, painful, or heavy periods, or lack of periods; anemia.

PSYCHOLOGICAL ASSOCIATIONS AND IMBALANCES: see the list on the left given for Stomach.

HEART

FUNCTION: awareness; our emotional center through which we interpret our environment; blood circulation.

PHYSICAL ASSOCIATIONS: heart organ; central nervous system; tongue and speech; sweat.

PHYSICAL IMBALANCES: heart disease and circulatory problems (usually more the province of the Heart Governor); palpitations; speech disorders; excessive sweating (often at night).

PSYCHOLOGICAL ASSOCIATIONS: Heart houses the Shen, which is the spirit and mind; consciousness, compassion; emotions; joy communication; sleep; long-term memory.

PSYCHOLOGICAL IMBALANCES: lack of compassion and empathy, mental restlessness; emotional instability, lack of emotion; hysteria; speech problems and inability to communicate; insomnia, dream-disturbed sleep; memory problems.

SMALL INTESTINE

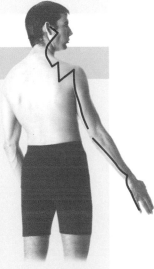

FUNCTION: assimilation; absorption of nutrients into the blood; separation of that which is useful to the body-mind from that which is not (classically known as "separating the pure from the impure").

PHYSICAL ASSOCIATIONS: small intestine, physical passage of nutrients from the digestive tract through the cell walls into the bloodstream.

PHYSICAL IMBALANCES: poor absorption of nutrients, intestinal gas, abdominal pain, anemia.

PSYCHOLOGICAL ASSOCIATIONS: clarity of judgment (separating one thing from another); dealing with mental anxiety, emotional excitement, and shock; determination.

PSYCHOLOGICAL IMBALANCES: inability to make decisions, cloudy judgment; inappropriate reaction to shock.

BLADDER

FUNCTION: purification; storage and excretion of urine.

PHYSICAL ASSOCIATIONS: urinary system; water metabolism; bones and teeth; head hair; ears; the spinal column; autonomic nervous system.

PHYSICAL IMBALANCES: any urinary problems including incontinence, urine retention, enlarged prostate; bone diseases including osteoporosis and some forms of arthritis; poor teeth; premature balding or gray hair; hearing problems and vertigo; lower back pain or weakness; overactivity of either sympathetic or parasympathetic division of the autonomic nervous system resulting in inappropriate reaction to stress, inability to relax, being too "laid back."

PSYCHOLOGICAL ASSOCIATIONS: fluidity; courage.

PSYCHOLOGICAL IMBALANCES: restlessness; fearfulness and timidity, recklessness.

KIDNEYS

FUNCTION: impetus; willpower and progress in life; governs reproduction and sexual activity; houses the Jing.

PHYSICAL ASSOCIATIONS: the kidneys; the endocrine system, hormones, the reproductive system; potential and pace of life; level of energy; water metabolism; ears; bones and teeth; lower back; genetic inheritance.

PHYSICAL IMBALANCES: kidney disorders; hormonal and endocrine disturbances, reproductive and sexual problems; irregularities in normal physical development; chronic tiredness; fluid retention and water metabolism problems; hearing and balance problems; weak bones and teeth; weakness, coldness or pain in the lower back; congenital and hereditary diseases.

PSYCHOLOGICAL ASSOCIATIONS: willpower, drive; ancestral Ki, genetic inheritance; courage; fluidity of emotions; short-term memory.

PSYCHOLOGICAL IMBALANCES: lack of determination and drive inherited psychological conditions; fear and phobias; restlessness; forgetfulness.

GALL BLADDER

FUNCTION: storage and distribution; bile; body movement; judgment.

PHYSICAL ASSOCIATIONS: gall bladder; sides of the body; joints, muscles, and tendons; digestion of fats; eyes.

PHYSICAL IMBALANCES: gall bladder problems; stiffness in movements; lack of bile; eye problems; stiffness in neck and shoulders, migraine; exhaustion.

PSYCHOLOGICAL ASSOCIATIONS: decision-making; creativity; good humor, irritability.

PSYCHOLOGICAL IMBALANCES: indecision; lack of creativity; overwork, attention to detail; frustration, impatience, constant irritation.

LIVER

FUNCTION: control; detoxification; storage; distribution; harmonizes emotions; plans.

PHYSICAL ASSOCIATIONS: storing and detoxifying blood; muscular system; eyes.

PHYSICAL IMBALANCES: any liver organ problem; menstrual problems; gout; tiredness; muscular pains, eye problems.

PSYCHOLOGICAL ASSOCIATIONS: control; planning; harmonious emotions; hardworking.

PSYCHOLOGICAL IMBALANCES: overcontrol or feeling of being out of control; excessive planning, inflexibility, frustration, repression; temper tantrums.

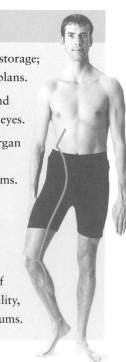

TRIPLE HEATER

FUNCTION: protection; harmonizes the generalized functions of the Upper, Middle, and Lower Heaters; the body's thermostat; protects the body's immunity via the lymphatic system; controls the opening of the waterways.

PHYSICAL ASSOCIATIONS: the Upper Heater is the heart and lungs regulating circulation and breathing, the Middle Heater is the stomach and spleen, dealing with digestion and transportation, the Lower Heater consists of kidney, bladder, liver, and small and large intestines, responsible for the separation of clean, usable fluid and food from the waste parts, which are then excreted; regulation of body temperature; lymphatic and immune system.

PHYSICAL IMBALANCES: lack of harmony between the three Heaters and their interrelated functions; poor heat regulation, poor circulation, overall chilliness or overheating; lymphatic problems, fluid and toxin retention; immune system disorders, allergies, lack of resistance to infections or illness.

PSYCHOLOGICAL ASSOCIATIONS: social interaction; emotional protection.

PSYCHOLOGICAL IMBALANCES: lack of warmth socially; overprotective or overprotected.

HEART GOVERNOR

FUNCTION: circulation; protects the heart.

PHYSICAL ASSOCIATIONS: the heart organ; arteries, veins; blood pressure.

PHYSICAL IMBALANCES: heart disease; circulatory disorders including hardening of the arteries, varicose veins, poor circulation; blood pressure disorders; tightness in the chest, angina, palpitations.

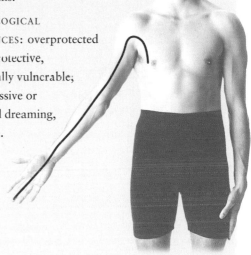

PSYCHOLOGICAL ASSOCIATIONS: protection of the emotions and the Shen; social relations; sleep and dreams.

PSYCHOLOGICAL IMBALANCES: overprotected or overprotective, emotionally vulnerable; shy; excessive or disturbed dreaming, insomnia.

THE TWO CENTRAL CHANNELS

In addition to the twelve bilateral meridians, there are two central channels.

CONCEPTION VESSEL

FUNCTION: influences all the Yin meridians; reproductive system.

ASSOCIATIONS: the abdomen, chest, lungs, throat and face; fertility, childbirth, menopause.

IMBALANCES: any reproductive problems, fibroids, lumps, hernia, coldness, weakness, lack of willpower.

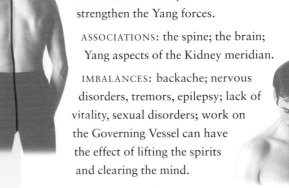

GOVERNING VESSEL

FUNCTION: influences all the Yang meridians in the body and can be used to strengthen the Yang forces.

ASSOCIATIONS: the spine; the brain; Yang aspects of the Kidney meridian.

IMBALANCES: backache; nervous disorders, tremors, epilepsy; lack of vitality, sexual disorders; work on the Governing Vessel can have the effect of lifting the spirits and clearing the mind.

5 Diagnosis

CHOOSING THE MERIDIAN

How does the practitioner decide which meridians to concentrate on during the session? If we were to use the meridian functions and associations purely in a symptomatic way, we might be able to choose a meridian or set of meridians to work on, but they might not be the most appropriate ones for the patient, either in the longer or the short term. What we use, therefore, is a framework of four methods of diagnosis in order to arrive at a conclusion about the patient's constitution (that is, his inherited and long-term tendencies), his condition (his short-term state of health), and a description of the Ki imbalance found. This last is summed up using whichever theory of Ki movement or dynamics the practitioner finds most applicable in practice. The most common theories used in Shiatsu diagnosis to describe what the Ki is actually doing are the Five Elements cycles, kyo-jitsu theory (from Zen Shiatsu), and the Eight Principles (these are used widely by traditional Chinese acupuncturists).

Before we look at these in a little more detail, let us examine the different forms of diagnosis used. There are four of these: asking questions, observation, hearing and smelling, and touch. All will probably be employed by the practitioner.

TOUCH DIAGNOSIS

The most commonly used method of touch diagnosis in Shiatsu is *hara diagnosis*. The hara has specific areas, which, when palpated, give feedback about the state of Ki in the meridian related to each. We use the hara because it tends to be relatively protected and hence gives a clear reading of the body's Ki status. In the same way, we have a map of the back with areas corresponding to meridians. There are also certain points on the front and back known as Bo points and Yu points, respectively, which when pressed may be tender or feel hard or soft; each of these is associated with an individual meridian.

Another method of touch diagnosis is using the pulses found on the radial artery; again there is a position for each of the meridians and the quality of the pulse tells the practitioner what is happening. Finally, there is the feel of the meridians themselves and how the Ki manifests in them.

THEORIES OF KI FLOW USED IN DIAGNOSIS

The diagnosis reached by the four forms can be explained using whichever theory of Ki flow the practitioner finds most appropriate. There are three major theories (see pp. 78–81).

FORMS OF DIAGNOSIS

Asking questions: which involves taking down a case history with details of a patient's current state of health along with finding out about his or her general personality, likes and dislikes, and so on.

Observation: noting general demeanor, posture, the colors of clothes, lines, features, and colors on the face. Observation would also include the intuitive feel picked up from patients.

Hearing and smelling: this refers to listening to the tone of voice patients use, whether sing-song, shouting, monotonous, weepy, or groaning (these are

Five Elements classifications). It also refers to the particular individual smells they give off, which has nothing to do with the aftershave or deodorant they wear. (I prefer my patients not to wear strongly perfumed products when they come for treatment, because they mask the individual's own personal scent, and also tend to be unpleasantly overpowering for people who are sensitive to smell.)

Touch: this is the most important diagnostic tool in Shiatsu. There are certain well-defined areas where the practitioner can feel the quality of Ki in the meridians very clearly.

HARA DIAGNOSIS MAP

LU = Lung	KD = Kidney	ST = Stomach	HT = Heart
LI = Large Intestine	BL = Bladder	GB = Gall Bladder	HG = Heart Governor
SI = Small Intestine	LIV = Liver	SP = Spleen	TH = Triple Heater

ABOVE *The Hara diagnosis map. A practitioner can feel the state of Ki in the meridian related to each area.*

THE YU POINTS

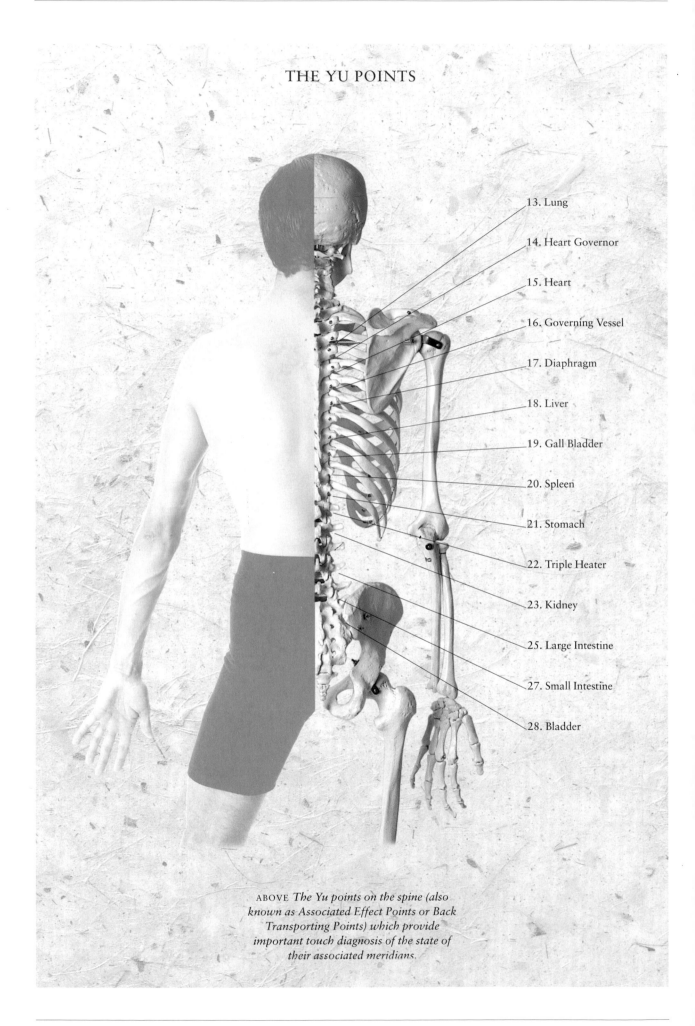

13. Lung

14. Heart Governor

15. Heart

16. Governing Vessel

17. Diaphragm

18. Liver

19. Gall Bladder

20. Spleen

21. Stomach

22. Triple Heater

23. Kidney

25. Large Intestine

27. Small Intestine

28. Bladder

ABOVE *The Yu points on the spine (also known as Associated Effect Points or Back Transporting Points) which provide important touch diagnosis of the state of their associated meridians.*

FIVE ELEMENT CASE HISTORY

Mrs. M., female, 36 years

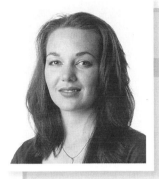

Mrs. M. arrived for her first treatment a little late and rather harassed since she had been busy dealing with details of her disabled daughter's transportation to a new school. Her principal health problem was evident; despite being only 36 years old, she had been suffering from painful rheumatoid arthritis for over 20 years. It had started in her left wrist and progressed to her elbows, ankles, and knees. The current attack was affecting mainly the right elbow, which was extremely painful and impossible to straighten. When we talked through her case history Mrs. M. was willing to look at the reasons underlying her condition. She felt that stress was a large factor in her problem.

In general her health was good; noteworthy features were indigestion, often due to eating too quickly, or to excessive use of aspirin for pain relief. She also had a tendency to feel chilly in all weathers especially in her hands, feet, and neck.

In terms of visual diagnosis Mrs. M. had a tendency to look quite red, with dark patches below her eyes or on either side of the bridge of the nose. This told me that Kidneys and Spleen were imbalanced and would need to be checked in hara.

In Traditional Chinese Medicine, rheumatoid arthritis is part of a group of conditions known as "painful obstruction syndrome," which can arise through invasion by the pathogenic factors of Damp, Cold, and Wind, or because of long-term emotional stagnation of Ki involving anger and resentment. Having taken her full case history I felt the condition was more of a chronic nature, with Damp being the major causative factor. Dampness in particular has a damaging effect on the Spleen, and as well as visual indications that all was not in balance with Spleen, her digestive difficulties and occasional feelings of low self esteem, combined with consistent activities to help everyone else but herself, pointed to depleted energy in Spleen.

When we got down to hara diagnosis the pattern for the first few sessions was Spleen kyo with either Gall Bladder or Liver jitsu. Using Masunaga's theory of Kyo-jitsu, Spleen kyo combined with Gall Bladder jitsu produces symptoms of incomplete digestion, restlessness, anxiety, and obsession with details, resulting in over-eating, brooding over things and arthritis in the knees. Mrs. M's tendency not to take time to digest things, either physically or mentally, was apparent at times, as was the tendency not to listen to her own body when it asked for rest. The Gall Bladder's function of distributing Ki and supporting Liver in governing smooth flow of Ki was thus compromised.

During the first sessions we concentrated on the areas of pain and stiffness, accessing them by the meridians showing most kyo and jitsu. In particular we used the supplementary channels for SP and GB in the arms to focus on her elbows and wrists, while spending time on specific points to tonify SP and dispel Dampness on the traditional SP meridian in the leg. Mrs. M commented that she felt good after her treatments, with lots more energy. However, the right elbow remained sore for quite some time. Recommendations included amending her diet to include more warming and drying foods, and a gentle exercise routine. Either yoga or tai chi would have been appropriate: she opted for a yoga class, but so far has not been a regular attender – part of the ongoing pattern of behavior sustaining the Ki imbalance.

Five Element Cycles

This refers to the Creative and Control cycles described earlier in the chapter. If Ki is balanced throughout the body-mind, it will flow smoothly around both cycles. If, however, it is disturbed anywhere, then blockages and weaknesses will occur in patterns that follow the Creative and Control cycles.

Here is a simple example. If someone has strong ambition and willpower (Water), he or she will tend to push themselves and overtax the autonomic nervous system, resulting in stress and inability to relax – this is an excessive Water condition. This excess is then pushed around the Creative cycle to the Wood element, where it may manifest as headaches, irritability, overwork, tendency to drink too much alcohol, and constant planning. Using the Control cycle, the excessive Wood would then typically restrain the Earth element too much, causing possible indigestion, stomach ulcers, and swings of high and low energy through the day – these are symptoms of low Earth energy. The Earth would have insufficient energy to control the Water and so the whole round would start again. Doesn't this sound like a typical overworked business person?

Of course, this is a relative simplification, since all the Elements would be involved since they are all related. Just as a stone dropped in a pool causes ripples over the whole surface, any Ki disturbance has repercussions throughout the whole body-mind.

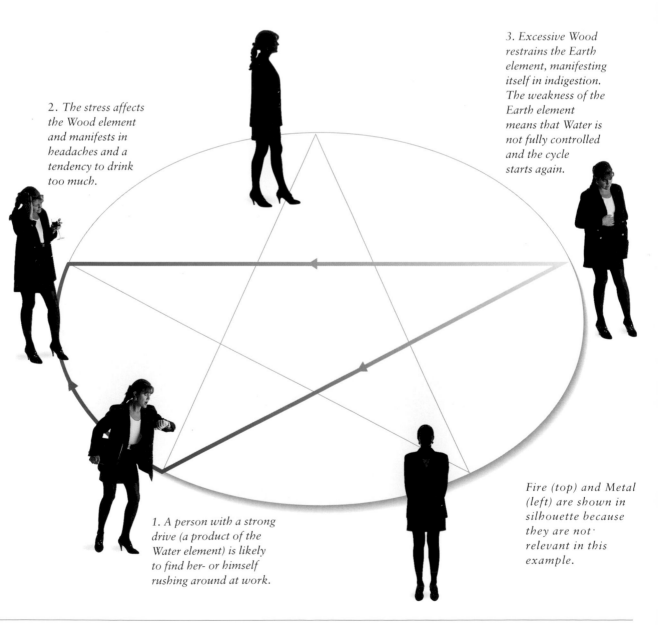

2. The stress affects the Wood element and manifests in headaches and a tendency to drink too much.

3. Excessive Wood restrains the Earth element, manifesting itself in indigestion. The weakness of the Earth element means that Water is not fully controlled and the cycle starts again.

1. A person with a strong drive (a product of the Water element) is likely to find her- or himself rushing around at work.

Fire (top) and Metal (left) are shown in silhouette because they are not relevant in this example.

CASE HISTORY USING FIVE ELEMENT THEORY

Mr. H., male, 39 years

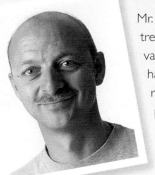

Mr. H's reasons for seeking treatment were a little vague and nonspecific. He had been experiencing recurrent colds over the previous six months, in combination with feelings of tiredness, and a general "lack of motivation." My initial visual diagnosis of a typical Metallic type (tall and fair with pale heart- shaped face, broad shoulders and slim hips, precise but slow way of moving) was confirmed on taking his case history, which revealed a background of eczema, constriction in the chest and nasal obstruction, along with a natural liking for order and method in his life.

Because the Metal dominance in Mr. H's case was so clear-cut, I decided to use the Five Element method of treatment both in the individual sessions and to stand back and review his entire case. Where Metal had originally been balanced, over the years the emotional and psychological aspects had become accentuated, causing a sense of isolation, and a certain sadness or melancholy at not being able to communicate with others effectively. This movement toward an excess condition had reversed after a bereavement, which left him depressed and hopeless. His job was quite intellectual with prolonged spells sitting at a desk in a centrally heated office: this had obviously been detrimental on a physical level, leading to the recurring colds. It seemed that Mr. H was suffering from a deficiency of Metal, and of Lung Ki, in that he was unable to breathe deeply and mobilize the energy in his chest, resulting in repeated colds, and tiredness.

Hara diagnosis over the series of sessions was interesting in that Lung or occasionally Large Intestine were the consistent deficient meridians (Kidney also manifested kyo on several occasions), but excess showed up at some time in all of the other Elements. Using the Five Element treatment method, I first tonified Lung and also Spleen in order to increase Lung energy. Working Spleen had several other

functions: it helped to drain energy from the excessive Heart meridian, and on a more specific level the tsubos SP6, SP9, and SP10 were helpful in combating a Damp Heat condition, which I felt was responsible for his chronic eczema. Secondly, I did a little intuitive tonifying work on the Kidney meridian in the legs, partly to balance the excessive Heart meridian and partly to increase his general level of energy.

In subsequent treatments both Bladder and Stomach came up jitsu along with Lung kyo and in one case Large Intestine kyo; later there was a pattern of Lung kyo and Gall Bladder jitsu. Since his energy was on the whole higher than when treatment began, in these sessions I was able to work with the Control cycle (as a principle of treatment, if energy is lacking it is good to mobilize the Creative cycle and if energy is high it is appropriate to use the Control cycle). The method was to tonify the deficiency in Lung, which also controled the excess in Gall Bladder. Some work was also done to sedate Gall Bladder, which helped with his digestive problems.

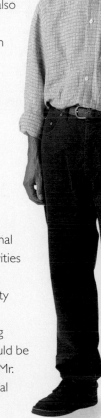

Treatment resulted in increased physical energy and more positivity. The chest constriction continued to be a problem, but breathing exercises and Qi Gong slowly bore fruit. On a psychological and emotional level I suggested that activities emphasizing the positive aspects of Wood (creativity and spontaneity) and Fire (being sociable, expressing emotions, having fun) would be of benefit to balance out Mr. H.'s longterm constitutional dominance in Metal.

Kyo-jitsu Theory

Masunaga's theory of kyo and jitsu illustrates the energetic distortion of Yin and Yang. Kyo is the more Yin quality; to the touch it feels either soft and empty, or stiff and resistant. Its overall characteristic is unresponsive. Jitsu on the other hand is more Yang in nature. It feels hard and full, bouncy and active.

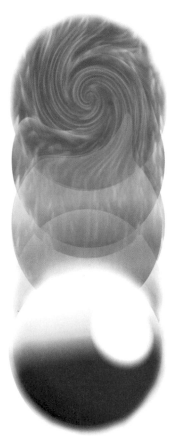

ABOVE *Kyo can be thought of as a deflated ball, soft and empty. Jitsu is hard and active, like an inflated ball.*

Its principal characteristic is responsive. Kyo and jitsu are always linked together in an energetic relationship in which the kyo causes the jitsu. The classic example of this is when we are hungry (empty and therefore kyo) we go off and find ourselves something to eat (activity, which is jitsu) and thus bring ourselves back to a comfortable balance. By working on the kyo, the cause or need, we can balance the jitsu. This system has a considerable amount of flexibility, since any meridian could be in an energetic relationship with another. However, it is rare to find meridians within the same Element in a kyo-jitsu relationship, because they have a similar Ki quality and therefore would not be both high and low in energy at the same time.

As an example of kyo-jitsu theory, let us imagine a person who has spent several years nursing a demanding elderly relative who has recently died. This person has expended a great deal of caring, compassion, and emotional energy in difficult circumstances, perhaps having to contend with the demands of his or her own growing family, too, resulting in an emptiness (kyo) in the Heart meridian. On the death of the relative, our patient finds he or she feels stuck and unable to express grief. Not only this, but the patient now feels unwilling to go out and meet people again after so much time at home, and to cap it all has developed constipation with occasional explosive diarrhea – all symptoms of a jitsu Large Intestine. Therefore, the energetic relationship here is Heart kyo, Large Intestine jitsu. The depletion of the emotional forces of the Heart result in an inability to express grief and in turn the inability to let go of the relative. Treatment would take the form of increasing the energy in the Heart, which would relax the Large Intestine and allow it to let go, solving both the emotional and physical problems.

You will notice that this is a more emotional and psychological example. This is because Zen Shiatsu tends to put an emphasis on the psycho-emotional causes of imbalance and acknowledge their close relationship with physical symptoms.

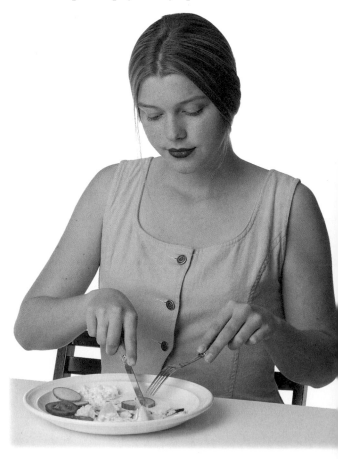

Eight Principles

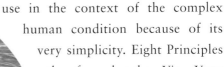

This is another way to describe and understand the patterns of Ki imbalance and is used extensively in the Traditional Chinese Medicine (T.C.M.) form of acupuncture. Some Shiatsu practitioners who are also acupuncturists make use of this theoretic model, although the technique that follows on from it is possibly more applicable to acupuncture and the specific action of points than to Shiatsu. The Eight Principles are Yin/Yang, Interior/Exterior, Empty/Full, and Cold/Hot. As we now know from the theory we have looked at so far, the six last categories are themselves subdivisions of Yin Yang. But again, as we have noted previously, the general theory of Yin Yang as applied to all phenomena is sometimes difficult to

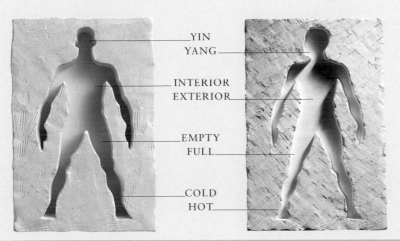

ABOVE *The Yin Yang theory accounts for all phenomena.*

use in the context of the complex human condition because of its very simplicity. Eight Principles therefore breaks Yin Yang down into more understandable parts to give a description of the energy state. It is interesting to note that in contrast to this, Five Element theory gives us more a description of energy movement or process of change.

Each of these theoretical systems provides the Shiatsu practitioner with the means to be able to sum up where Ki may be distorted, and this in turn shows the means to treat the imbalance. It should be noted that these are all theories; in other words, descriptions of reality – it is the practitioner's job to be able to use theory to fit reality, not to try to squeeze reality into a theory.

EIGHT PRINCIPLES

Interior/Exterior describes the location of the imbalance.

Empty/Full indicates whether Ki is deficient (similar to kyo), with chronic symptoms, weakness, tiredness, inactivity, and pain helped by pressure; or excessive (jitsu), with acute conditions involving restlessness, heavy breathing, and pain on pressure.

Cold/Hot refers to the nature of the symptoms, with Cold conditions resulting in feeling cold, pale face, no thirst, and Hot in overheating, fever, red face, thirst, and constipation.

Yin/Yang refers to the overall Yin Yang balance and to specific tendencies when imbalanced. For instance, Yin tendencies would include being weak and tired, feeling cold, wanting to keep warm, lack of appetite, wanting to be held or touched, while Yang signs include activity, restlessness, feeling hot, thirst, and finding pressure or touch painful.

YIN
YANG
INTERIOR
EXTERIOR
EMPTY
FULL
COLD
HOT

LEFT *The sets of opposites in the human body.*

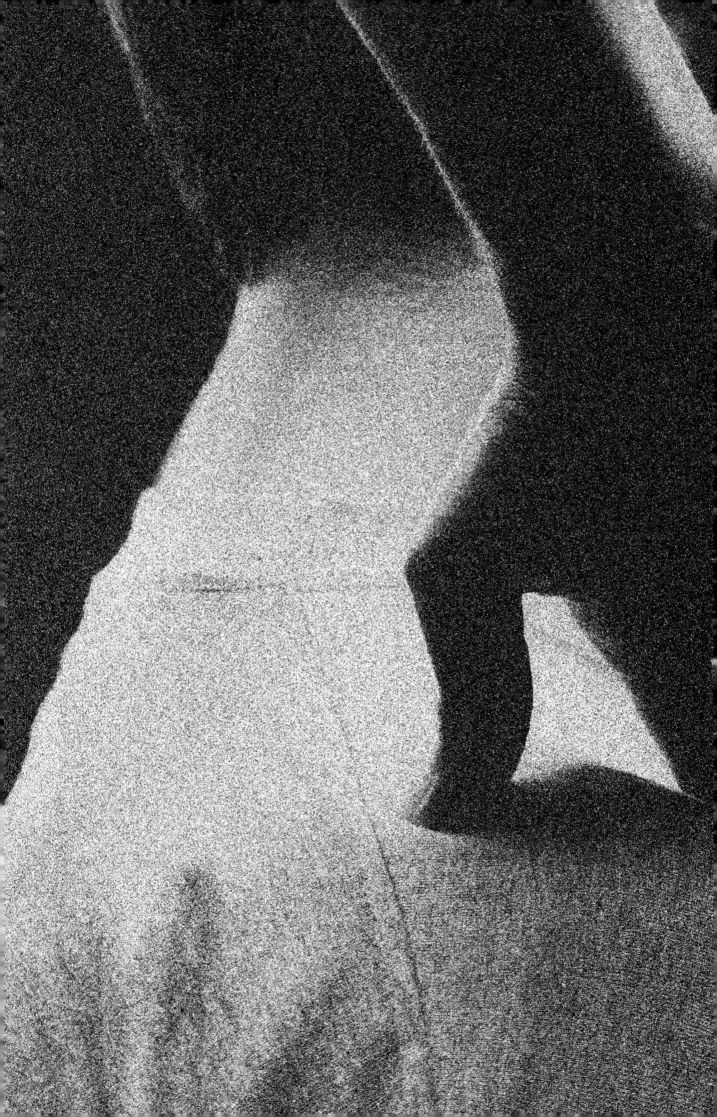

THE TECHNIQUES OF SHIATSU

Shiatsu technique involves the whole body, but mainly the hands, which act not only as the instruments of pressure but also as sensitive probes of the patient's condition.

1 Application of Technique

Now that we have arrived at a diagnosis, a description of the Ki imbalance, what do we do about it? This is where we start to apply the techniques of Shiatsu. Our hands are our primary tools, but in order for them to be used sensitively, they must be comfortable. Having a relaxed, open posture allows you to focus your attention on your hands and what they are feeling, so it is important to position yourself in such a way that you can reach the part of the body you are working on without any strain or discomfort. An aid to this is always to remember to have your work in front of you, preferably close to your hara, your seat of power. A further tip is to have a fairly wide stance, with knees or knee and foot sufficiently far apart to give you a stable, balanced base to work from.

Working with two hands is a feature of Zen Shiatsu, and not only enables the practitioner to monitor his or her partner's Ki more easily, but also feels more supportive to the receiver. "Two-handed" techniques may involve two thumbs, palm and thumb, knee and thumb, and so on. Because we are in contact with the body throughout the treatment, we are going to be getting a lot of tactile feedback. I like to encourage my students to describe what they are feeling in creative or imaginative ways. This helps them to concentrate on the exact feel they are getting. In reading texts on Shiatsu and other forms of oriental medicine we tend to come across standard terms, such as "excessive" or "deficient," which are useful as a starting point, but can limit our perception of touch if we stick rigidly to them.

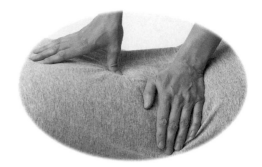

ABOVE *The palm and thumb technique.*

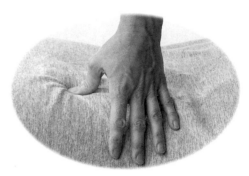

ABOVE *Using one thumb only. The fingers provide rest and stability.*

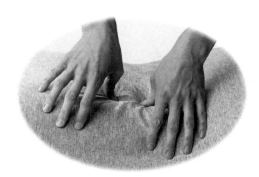

ABOVE *Using two thumbs for two-handed techniques.*

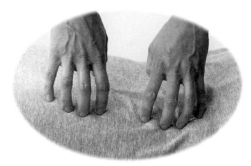

ABOVE *The two-handed technique using all the fingers.*

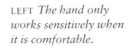

LEFT *The hand only works sensitively when it is comfortable.*

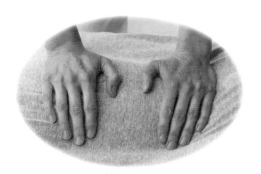

ABOVE *Using both palms for deeper pressure.*

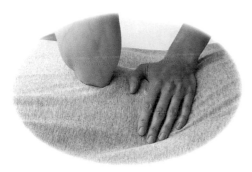

ABOVE *Using the elbow can be a less tiring way of applying pressure.*

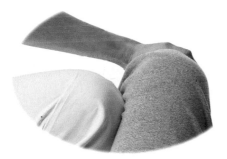

ABOVE *The knee provides stability for some treatments.*

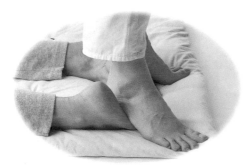

ABOVE *Standing techniques involving foot to foot contact may be used.*

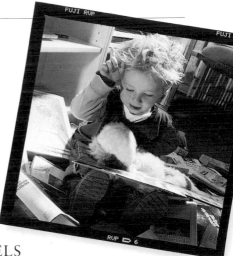

RIGHT *Shiatsu has been found especially helpful in dealing with hyperactivity in children, because it directs and controls wayward energies.*

HOW KYO FEELS

In speaking of kyo we can say it is essentially unresponsive; in practice it may feel soft, like Jello, a sinking feeling, nothing there to hold you out, or stiff, like a creaky board, with no "give" to it. Because the feeling in terms of quantity is "not enough," we deal with kyo by putting more energy into the meridian, a process known as "tonification." This is effected by long, slow, holding pressure at medium-to-light depth, although always deep enough to contact the Ki. As a practitioner you can either hold passively and allow the receiver's Ki to focus into the point and fill it up, or you can consciously extend your own Ki into that tsubo using the hara and breathing techniques. The receiver will feel the sensation of your reaching and moving Ki in a kyo tsubo as a "nice pain," a comforting pressure that feels supportive.

HOW JITSU FEELS

Jitsu is classically described as hard or responsive, but more creatively, we may pick it up as bounding, bouncy, not letting you in, holding out, stuck, or stagnant. In terms of quantity, jitsu has too much Ki, so we want to encourage it to move on elsewhere by "sedation." Usually, in the ordinary way of speaking, to sedate someone would make us think of putting him or her to sleep, but in this case a better image is calming a hyperactive child to bring it back to a normal level of activity. Sedation techniques are fast, strong, and deep, and may be painful if applied to a site of long-term stagnation.

Being able to feel these different qualities is something that comes with practice. Two aids to sensitivity and intuition used in Shiatsu are the use of the hara and breathing.

The Hara

The abdomen, known as the hara, has great importance in Japanese culture and the Eastern understanding of the Self. In the West we tend to think of ourselves in terms of our mind and our brain, with the body tacked on as an appendage. The oriental viewpoint puts the center of ourself in the hara, with our vital energies, our seat of power and our intuitive faculties all based in this essential area. Although we talk about "having a gut feeling" about something, or "not having the guts" to do something, the Japanese concept of living and working from hara is very much wider than anything similar found in the West.

Most of us are familiar with the feats of martial artists, breaking through multiple blocks of wood or throwing someone of weighty proportions to the ground. This is done by using the hara as a power center and the effects can easily be seen. But the faculties of hara are also used in other Japanese arts: where to place a bloom in flower arranging or when to make the final brush stroke in a work of calligraphy. Using hara encompasses within it the idea of seeking perfection, or even enlightenment, through disciplined practice. There is no competitive element, for this is an inner, spiritual way. Developing the use of hara can be accomplished through many different media: meditation, exercise, martial arts, and, of course, Shiatsu.

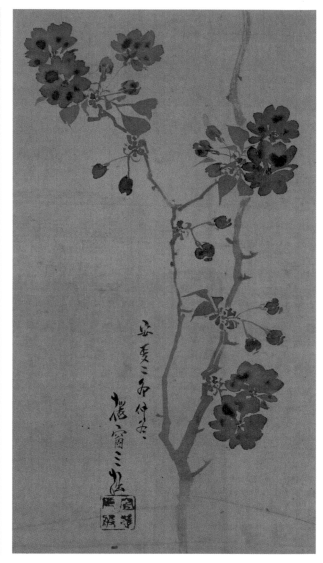

ABOVE *Hara is the source of esthetic judgment as well as strength.*

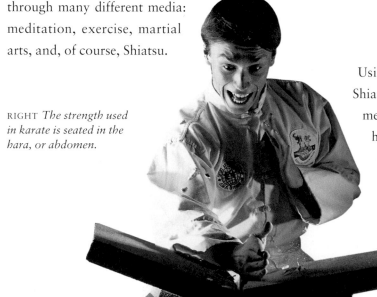

RIGHT *The strength used in karate is seated in the hara, or abdomen.*

Using the power and sensitivity of hara gives Shiatsu practitioners the capacity to move beyond mere technique to powerful and compassionate healing in the largest sense of the word. Being based in hara increases our intuition and the sensitivity we have in our hands; it enables us to empathize with the receiver sufficiently to feel what they are feeling, yet gives us the distance not to be caught up in their problems and their symptoms. Some simple exercises to help you get in touch with your own hara are included on pages 142 and 143.

Breathing

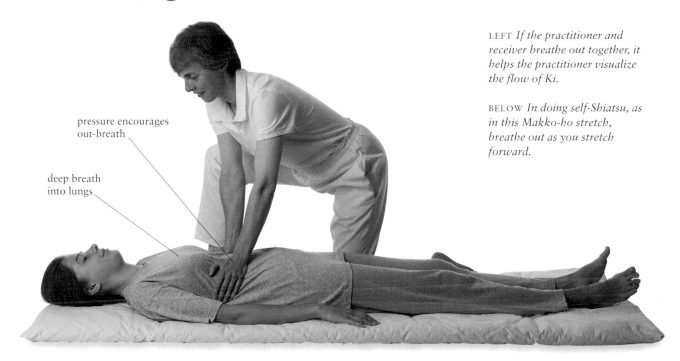

pressure encourages
out-breath

deep breath
into lungs

U se of the breath is another helpful tool in making Shiatsu more effective. The breath is in fact one of the most powerful tools at our disposal in life. If we breathe deeply we energize ourselves and accept life to the full; if our breathing is shallow we lack vitality, almost a negation of being here at all. Inhalation fills us with new, clean Ki, energizing our entire system. Exhalation is the powerful and relaxing breath that allows us to relax and reach out to life. We all know that we sigh with relief, or to let go of old feelings, but we

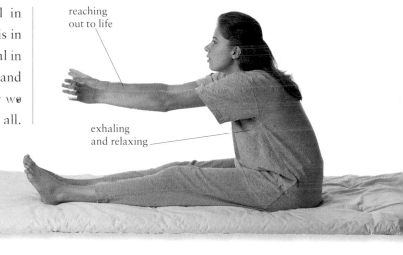

reaching
out to life

exhaling
and relaxing

may be less in touch with the powerful aspect of breathing out. Next time you are trying to undo a stuck jam jar, do it while breathing out and you will be surprised at the results! In Shiatsu we tend to apply pressure when we are breathing out and when the receiver is exhaling, too. This allows us to visualize the flow of Ki through our hands more easily, and the receiver can relax and let go of any tension. By coordinating breathing in this way we can feel closer to each other and this empathy encourages the healing process.

The easiest way to get in touch with our breathing is to visualize the breath going down to the hara.

Although obviously when we breathe in, it is our physical lungs that fill, by imagining our breath deepening down and filling the abdomen we have a powerful sense of being filled with strength. As a preliminary to giving Shiatsu, a practitioner will often spend a few minutes practicing hara breathing. In this dynamic meditation technique, we visualize the air as a stream of light filling up the hara; the out breath is quiet and long, allowing the Ki to settle and remain at the tanden. After several breaths we have a sense of warmth and of gathering a store of Ki at our center: this centered feeling can then be taken into the treatment.

② Tsubo: the Classical Acupuncture Points

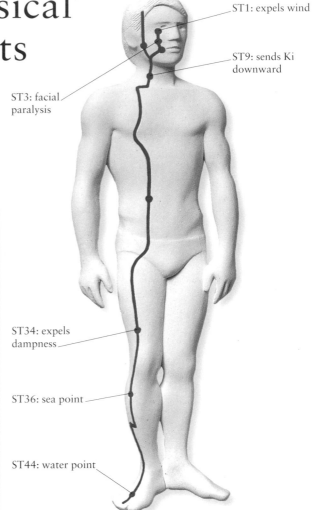

ST1: expels wind

ST9: sends Ki downward

ST3: facial paralysis

ST34: expels dampness

ST36: sea point

ST44: water point

ABOVE *Each tsubo on a meridian has a specific function as well as balancing the overall energy of the channel.*

The tsubo or classical acupuncture points are places where Ki accumulates on the meridians, like pools in a stream, and here it is easier to tap into Ki and manipulate it. The tsubo are numbered according to their position on the meridian: for example, KD1 is the first tsubo on the Kidney meridian. Points also have poetic names, which give an indication of their location or their uses; for example ST1, "Containing Tears," is located on the lower eye socket just below the eye, and one of its functions is to stop excessive watering.

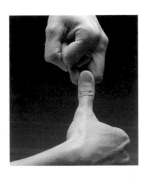

ABOVE *Tsubo are located by proportional measurements called "cun." One cun is the distance between the two creases on the middle fingers, roughly one thumb's width.*

Modern scientific investigation has shown that the classical points are often situated at places where there are particular physical features: for example, around joints, in the depressions between muscles, or where nerves run superficially. The electrical resistance of the skin at these points can be measured using electronic equipment and has been demonstrated to be lower than elsewhere on the body's surface. This points conclusively to the fact that something is going on there, even if orthodox medicine has not yet managed to define the exact nature of that "something."

THE PROPERTIES OF TSUBO

Each classical tsubo has specific properties or actions. These may include reducing pain, moving Ki in specific directions, calming the mind, heating or cooling the body, or balancing the Elements. Points on the hands as far as the elbow, and on the feet as far as the knee, tend to be more dynamic than other more central tsubo, since here the Ki is nearer the surface and so more easily affected.

Another interesting aspect of the use of points is the fact that they can be used for diagnostic purposes. On the back, a series of points running down the Bladder meridian known in Japanese as the Yu points (Associated Effect or Back Transporting points) can be palpated to diagnose the state of each of the internal organs. These particular points correlate very approximately with the locations of autonomic nervous system pathways exiting the spinal column and feeding the corresponding organs. Bo points (Front Collecting points) are located on the midline (Conception Vessel) or at specific tsubo on the ribcage, and again correspond to the state of meridian energy in particular organs. Sharp pain or tenderness on pressure on either Yu or Bo points

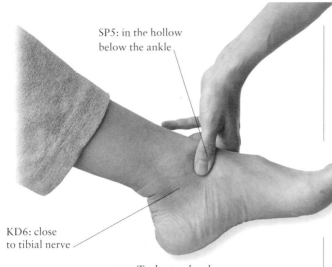

SP5: in the hollow
below the ankle

KD6: close
to tibial nerve

ABOVE *Tsubo tend to be
located at joints, between
muscles, or near nerves.*

From the point of view of energy, a tsubo is shaped like a vase with a narrow neck and wide belly. In order to contact the Ki contained in the point, you must direct pressure in at 90 degrees to the skin surface. By being precise about perpendicular pressure, being grounded in hara, and working into the tsubo with relaxed hands and arms, the Ki in the tsubo can be felt more clearly. Tsubo can be found anywhere on a meridian; the Shiatsu practitioner's task is to find which need attention and apply the appropriate technique. Does the tsubo feel empty and unresponsive? In that case it is kyo and needs to be tonified, encouraged to fill up, with long, slow holding. If a tsubo feels tight and full it is expressing a more jitsu quality and may need to be sedated with faster, more dynamic pressure. By evening out the feel in individual tsubo, the whole meridian is balanced and reintegrated into the body's energetic system.

As well as points on the meridians, other areas may become spontaneously painful; these are known as *Ahshi* or "ouch" points because people say "ouch" when they are pressed. They are areas where the skin and underlying muscle have become extra sensitive, often through chronic tightness. These jitsu areas can be dispersed with pressure techniques.

Within a Shiatsu session there is normally a balance between work on classic points (for their specific functions), on Ahshi points to relieve areas of particular tension, and work on imbalanced tsubo found on the meridians chosen for that session.

coupled with a hard sensation denotes an excess of energy in that meridian or organ, while a dull ache and feeling of softness or lack of response means Ki is lacking in the related meridian.

USING TSUBO IN SHIATSU

The theory of the action of points is obviously widely used in acupuncture. In Shiatsu, tsubo can be useful for first aid or specific symptoms, or as a diagnostic tool. However, in Zen Shiatsu, we tend to work more with the meridian energy, feeling by intuition and sensitivity where the Ki disturbances are and working accordingly. In this sense we are not working with the classical tsubo (although a knowledge of their whereabouts and functions is essential), but are feeling out for anywhere on a meridian where Ki may be distorted.

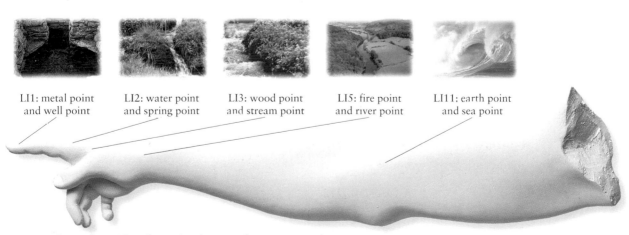

LI1: metal point
and well point

LI2: water point
and spring point

LI3: wood point
and stream point

LI5: fire point
and river point

LI11: earth point
and sea point

ABOVE *On each meridian five points between fingers (or toes for leg meridians) and elbows (or knees) are designated as the Five Element points. They have similar properties to a water course.*

The Physiology of Shiatsu

Having looked at how Shiatsu works from a purely oriental point of view, it is perhaps useful to consider the scientific explanations which, to our analytical and logical minds, provide the answer to how Shiatsu works on a material level. Much of the research work that has been done on the effects of acupuncture, massage, and meditation can be applied to the *modus operandi* of Shiatsu. A knowledge of some of the body's physiological workings is helpful in explaining Shiatsu's undoubted effectiveness.

NERVE REFLEX ACTIONS

Research by Katsusuke Serizawa has established that the internal organs are linked to the skin, subcutaneous tissues, and muscles via the nervous system, and that by means of nerve reflex actions, disturbances in the functioning of the internal organs can be felt on the surface of the body. His research has verified that the reverse is also true: that by stimulating a tsubo close to the spinal column corresponding to a particular spinal nerve, a reflex action is set up and the functioning of the organ fed by that nerve can be enhanced.

NERVE REPORTING STATIONS

Very often when patients come for Shiatsu treatment, it is because they are experiencing pain, often of a long-term or chronic nature, and they are unhappy about the long-term use of pain-killing drugs that mask symptoms rather than deal with the underlying causes. By understanding how the nervous system works we can see why the role of pressure is important in pain control. Pain is very often caused by chronic and inappropriate tension in the muscles. Without going into too much detail, let us say that there are nerve reporting stations that fire off messages to the central nervous system about the length of muscle fibers and the load being carried by them. Sometimes, due to habitual movements, poor posture, or emotional tension, the reporting stations keep sending the message "hold on" even when the

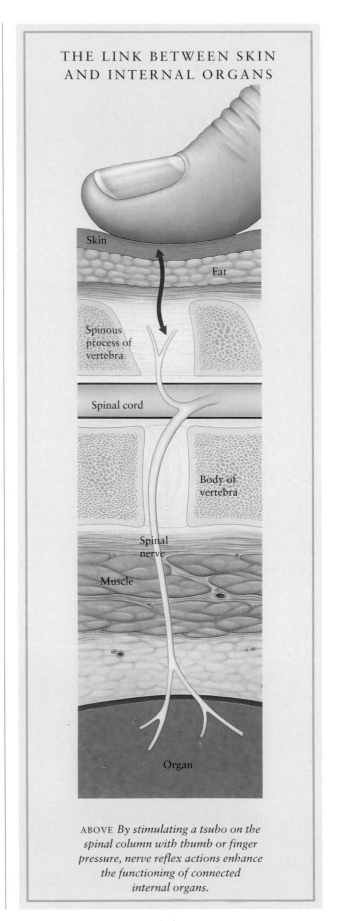

THE LINK BETWEEN SKIN AND INTERNAL ORGANS

Skin

Fat

Spinous process of vertebra

Spinal cord

Body of vertebra

Spinal nerve

Muscle

Organ

ABOVE *By stimulating a tsubo on the spinal column with thumb or finger pressure, nerve reflex actions enhance the functioning of connected internal organs.*

reason for the original muscle action is no longer there. A very simple example is the woman who always carries a shoulder bag on one side. On looking at her we find that one shoulder is higher than the other because the muscles have become so accustomed to the constant tension needed to hold up the weight of the bag that she has forgotten to let go of it when the bag has been put down.

TRIGGER POINTS

On working on her affected shoulder, the practitioner will find points that are extremely tender, which may refer pain up into her neck and head. These points are known as trigger points and can be equated with Ahshi points – the spontaneously arising painful tsubo acknowledged by Traditional Chinese Medicine. Pressure on trigger points will have two major effects. Firstly, it will displace the fluids concentrated in her overly contracted muscles and thus clear away toxic waste materials (such as lactic acid, which can cause cramp), which may have been contributing to the pain. The lymphatic system, which is responsible for draining toxins from the cells, will be activated, as will local circulation. With the increased capacity of the capilliaries in the area, fresh oxygenated blood will flow into the muscle cells, helping to further reduce the effects of any pain-inducing toxins.

THE GOLGI TENDON ORGANS

The second aspect of the effectiveness of pressure involves the workings of the central nervous system. The C.N.S. (the brain and spinal cord) is, briefly, responsible for receiving sensory information from our eyes, ears, and other sense organs, and in terms of our physical structures, lets us know, for example, which of our muscles is contracting and how quickly, the position and rate of movement of joints, and so on. As mentioned

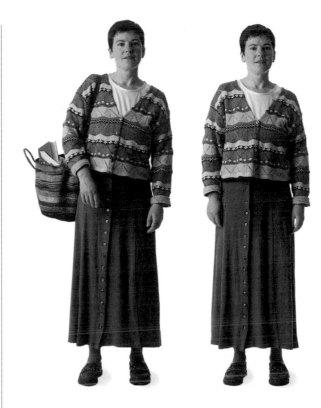

ABOVE *A habit, like always carrying a bag over the same shoulder, can fix muscles in a position even when it is not necessary.*

above, certain reporting stations in and around joints fire off messages to the C.N.S.; of these, the Golgi Tendon Organs are particularly interesting to us, since they measure the tension or load being born by muscle fibers. If the tendon organ detects an excess load or tension in the muscle, it may (in order to prevent tissue damage) relay messages telling the muscle to cease working, and relaxation of the muscle results. Pressure techniques and stretching used in Shiatsu have a direct effect on Golgi Tendon Organs, and thus our lady with her tense and sore shoulder will experience relief of her symptoms due to the workings of the nervous system.

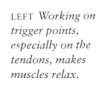

LEFT *Working on trigger points, especially on the tendons, makes muscles relax.*

▣ The Autonomic Nervous System

Finally, in looking at the calming and relaxing effect of Shiatsu overall, we must acknowledge the role of the autonomic nervous system (A.N.S.). The A.N.S. deals with the nervous functions that are not normally under our conscious control, such as the beating of the heart muscle and the contraction of muscles needed to move food along the digestive tract. This is in contrast to the C.N.S. (central nervous system) which deals with more conscious functions, such as the voluntary movement of skeletal muscle. The two divisions of the A.N.S. work together to govern our response to our surroundings, and activity between the two is usually balanced.

The *sympathetic* division of the A.N.S. deals with the "fight or flight" reaction, in which our body is geared up for stress: it stimulates the secretion of adrenalin, increasing heartbeat, opening air passageways, and widening the blood vessels supplying the muscles, while closing down on digestive and reproductive functions. The *parasympathetic* division reverses the effects of the sympathetic division, allowing the body to conserve and store energy, particularly through the increased activity of the digestive organs. The comforting, supportive, and pleasurable touch given in Shiatsu induces the activities of the parasympathetic division of the

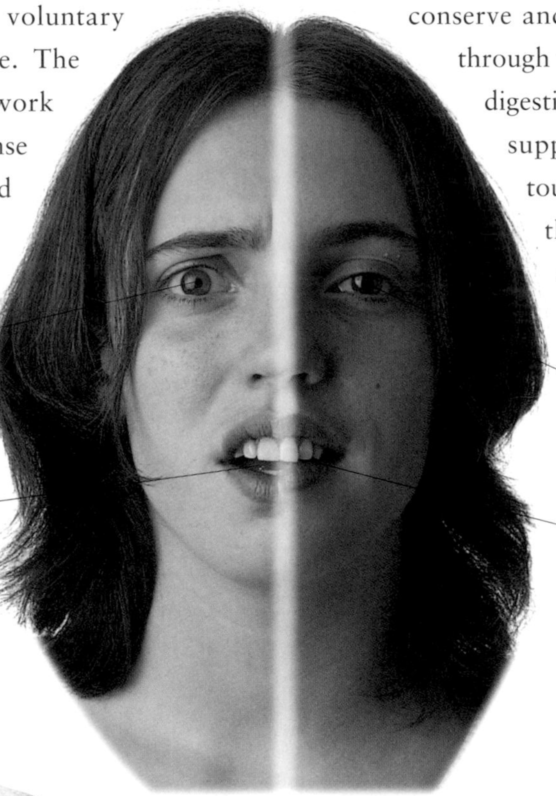

pupil dilates

pupil contracts

mouth is dry

stimulates salivation

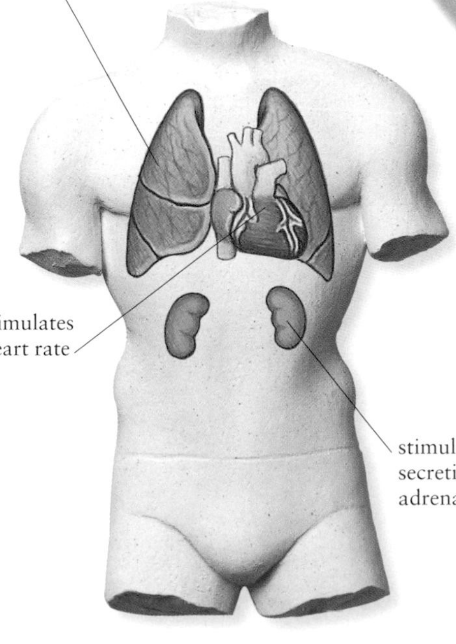

dilates bronchi

constricts bronchi

ABOVE *The autonomic nervous system is responsible for our automatic reactions to the environment. The sympathetic division is the "fright or flight" mechanism, whereas the parasympathetic division allows us to relax.*

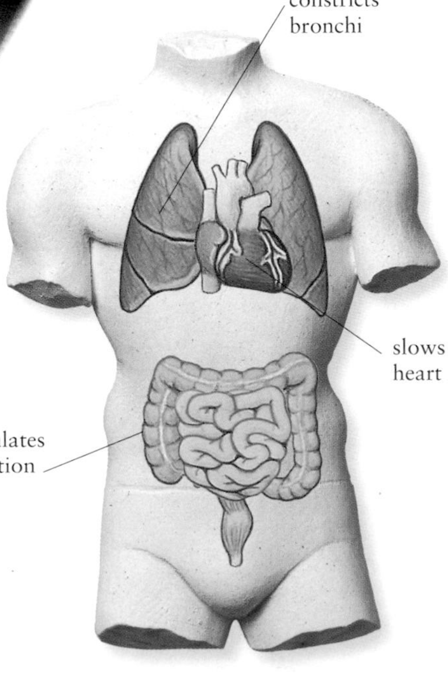

stimulates heart rate

slows heart rate

stimulates secretion of adrenalin

stimulates digestion

SYMPATHETIC DIVISION

PARASYMPATHETIC DIVISION

A.N.S. to predominate, resulting in overall relaxation, calmness, and a feeling of tranquility.

The nerve pathways of the sympathetic division lie mostly in the thoracic area of the spine, while those of the parasympathetic are located in the neck at the base of the skull and in the sacrum. Pressure on the Bladder (BL) meridian, which runs close to the spinal column from the head through the sacrum (the flat bone at the base of the spine), helps to normalize and synchronize the workings of both divisions of the A.N.S.

THE EFFECT OF ENDORPHINS

Another physiological explanation for the pain-relieving qualities of Shiatsu is the secretion of endorphins (endogenous morphines). Endorphins are neuropeptides (chemical messengers) within the brain with morphine-like properties, which act as natural analgesics, suppressing pain as well as regulating the body's response to stress and determining mood. "Runner's" or "swimmer's high" is thought to be the result of the release of endorphins during physical exertion. Research into acupuncture and massage has shown that they both stimulate the secretion of endorphins and, since Shiatsu combines aspects of both these therapies, it is highly likely that the techniques involved will also stimulate the body to release these natural painkillers. This is especially helpful for athletes or dancers, whose livelihood depends on their ability to overcome physical pain in the course of their daily training, competitions, or performances. It is also useful for pregnant women in labor, who can use Shiatsu techniques to help them with the pain of uterine contractions and thereby possibly avoid the necessity for artificial or chemical methods of pain relief.

THE IMPORTANCE OF SENSORY STIMULATION

We must not forget the importance of pleasant sensations when we talk of well-being. Sensory stimulation is vital to human well-being; babies can die from lack of physical contact; older people can feel cut off from the world, from themselves, and, in consequence, fade away slowly for lack of human contact. It is interesting that there are more pathways sending touch

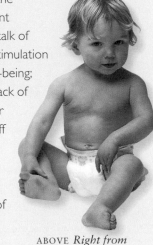

ABOVE *Right from babyhood we need sensory stimulation.*

sensation to the brain than those sending pain sensations. By creating pleasant tactile sensations away from the site of pain, we may distract the brain and thus diminish the effects of pain. Perhaps we could say the same on a wider scale: that by reaching out and touching someone in a caring and compassionate way we can lessen whatever pain is in his or her life and put a sense of well-being back in the forefront of the

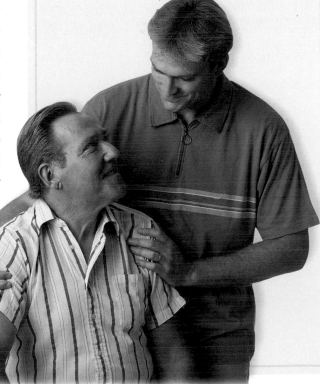

RIGHT *Any comforting touch or embrace stimulates the parasympathetic division.*

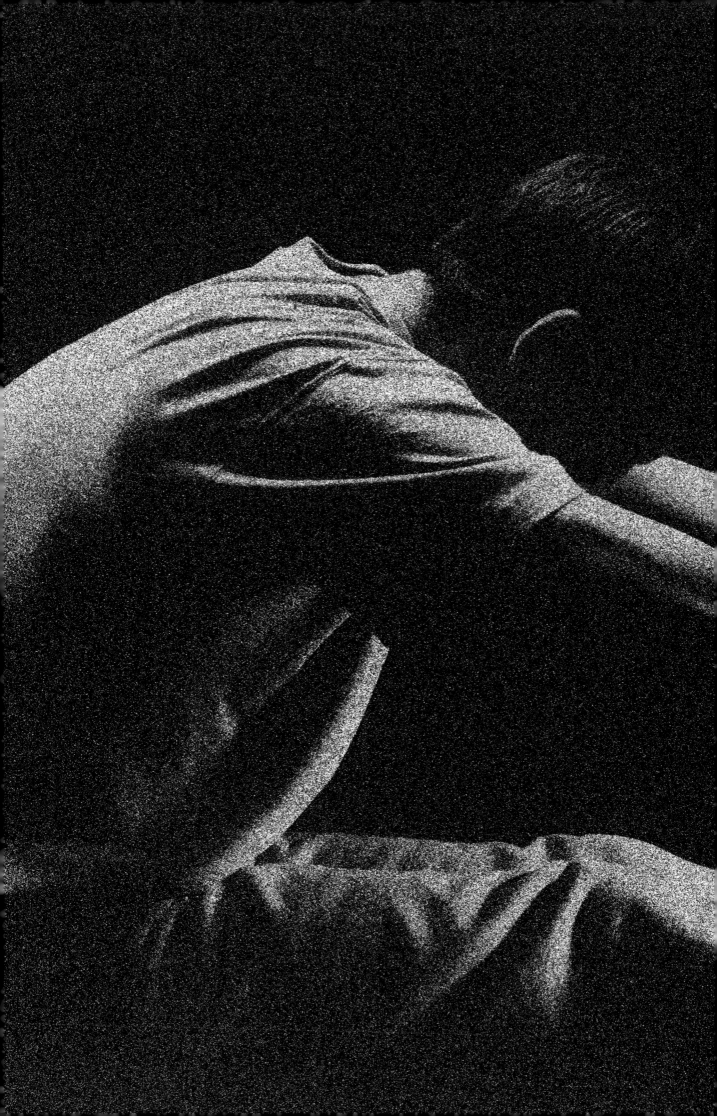

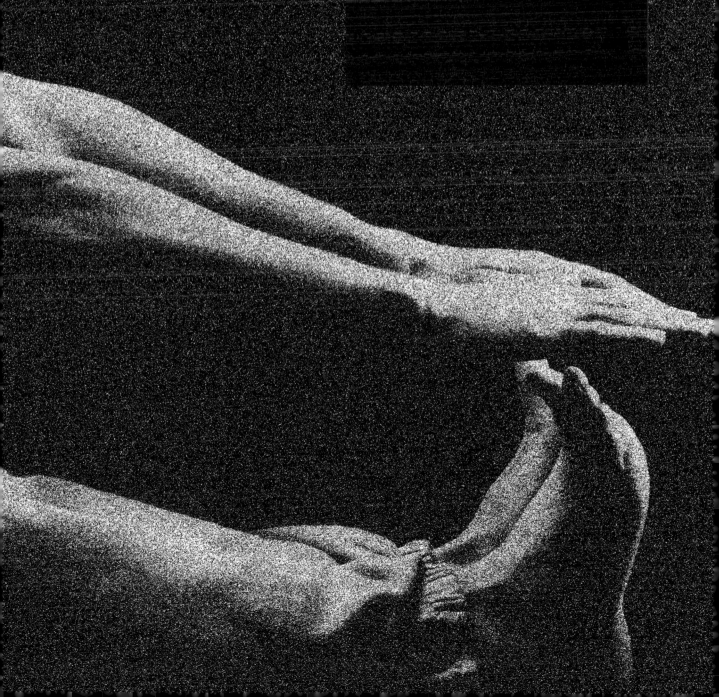

THE SHIATSU SEQUENCE

The Basic Sequence introduces the fundamentals of Shiatsu practice over the whole body, in a routine that can be applied beneficially to almost everyone.

1 Preparing Yourself as a Practitioner

The Basic Sequence outlined in this section is similar to the one that I teach my beginner students. It is a fairly simple routine, designed to stimulate all the meridians, to promote relaxation, and to ease out many of the everyday aches and pains that we are all prone to from time to time. Being a generalized treatment, it is quite appropriate for most people, so once you have mastered it you can practice it on your family and friends. Later in the book there are descriptions of advanced and specialized techniques, but I would encourage those of you who are fired with curiosity and enthusiasm by doing the Basic Sequence to go to Shiatsu classes, where you can learn more techniques and diagnosis.

One of my teachers once advised students to do 500 basic treatments before thinking of going on to more advanced ways of working, and using hara diagnosis and specific meridians. In many ways, I think this is sound advice. By practicing the basics until they become second nature, you become sufficiently confident not to have to worry about what to do next; at that point you can start to concentrate on how you are working and what you are feeling, and that is the time to start looking at more specific advanced work.

For those of you who do want to take a look at diagnosis, I have included a short section on how to do a simplified form of hara diagnosis after the Basic Sequence. Learning to do proper two-handed hara palpation really requires the presence of an experienced teacher to guide you through the various steps and to help you interpret what you are feeling. However, using the simplified form, along with the tables of meridian functions and associations (see pp. 70–73), can help you to pinpoint any imbalances. You can then concentrate on the relevant meridians within the context of this basic routine to make a more specific treatment for a particular condition.

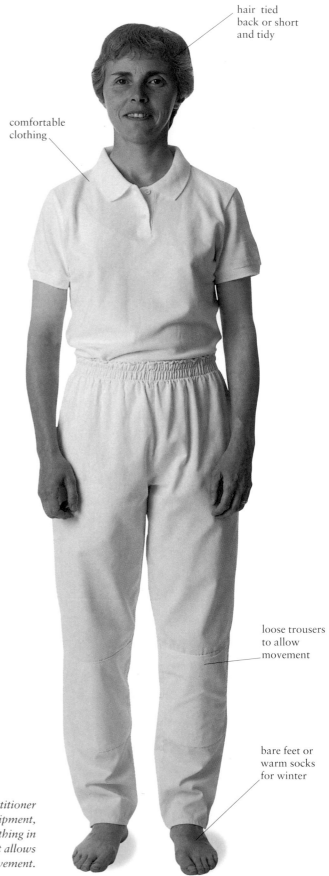

hair tied back or short and tidy

comfortable clothing

loose trousers to allow movement

bare feet or warm socks for winter

RIGHT *A shiatsu practitioner needs no special equipment, just comfortable clothing in neutral colors that allows freedom of movement.*

BELOW *Short sleeves allow the arms to move freely. Some practitioners practice barefoot, as left, others prefer to remain shod.*

RIGHT *Meridian "maps" to which the practitioner may refer for confirmation during diagnosis.*

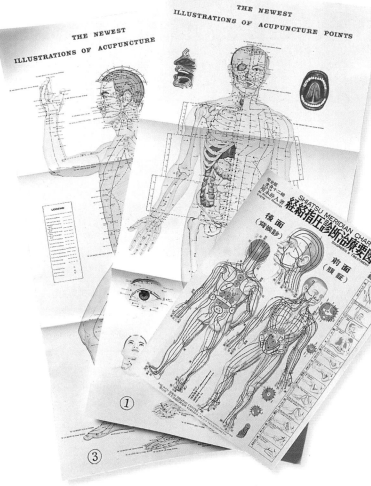

tidy haircut

comfortable tee shirt or sweater

sweat pants are ideal

shoes only if working on seated clients

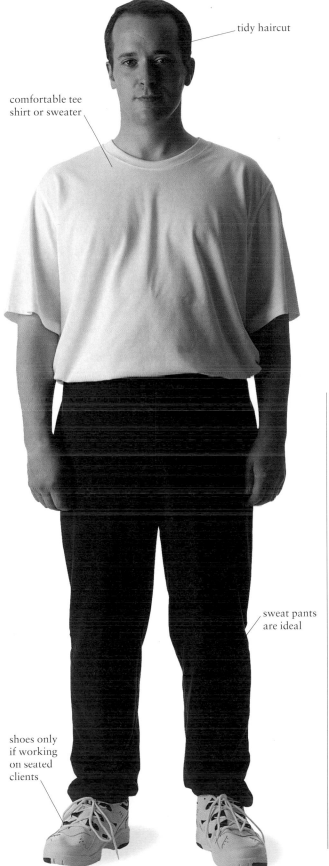

As a preparation for giving your first Shiatsu treatments, I would suggest reading through the Basic Sequence several times, to familiarize yourself with the overall structure of the session. In addition to studying the location of meridians as outlined on pages 70 to 73, detailed meridian charts, like those depicted above, are a useful learning tool to assist you with precise anatomical locations. Shiatsu and acupuncture schools often use three-dimensional models as teaching aids since these illustrate meridian flows more clearly.

In the end, however, reading and studying are no substitution for doing; so begin with your physical and mental preparations, then, to use a Zen phrase, "don't think, do it!"

RIGHT *Meridian charts (as top), or models showing the meridians and points, are useful learning aids.*

Preparing Your Body

Good preparation is the foundation of success in any activity, and Shiatsu is no exception. Except for the logistics of having the right room setting and timing, and the right attitude, of which more later, your own physical preparations are of great importance.

Being comfortable working and moving at floor level necessitates a certain suppleness and flexibility. Practice sitting in seiza (see p. 44) whenever you can, and when you get up and sit down, remember always to move from hara. Developing awareness of hara can be carried over to other activities in life: you will feel safer driving in heavy traffic in hara, moving large or difficult loads is less of a strain if you carry from hara, and, having recently begun horse riding, I find that keeping in command of my headstrong young horse is easier if I stay down in hara.

EXTENDING KI THROUGH YOUR HANDS

Hara breathing allows you to center your own Ki in readiness for giving Shiatsu (you will find some hara development exercises on pages 142–3). One final exercise that is useful preparation before a session is to extend Ki through your hands.

◎ Sit in seiza (see p. 44) with your hands resting, palm upward, on your knees. Breathe into hara, and on each out breath, visualize Ki flowing from hara through your shoulders and arms and out through your palms.

◎ A variation is to hold your palms about three inches apart and do the same exercise. You should notice a feeling of warmth as your hands become charged up with Ki.

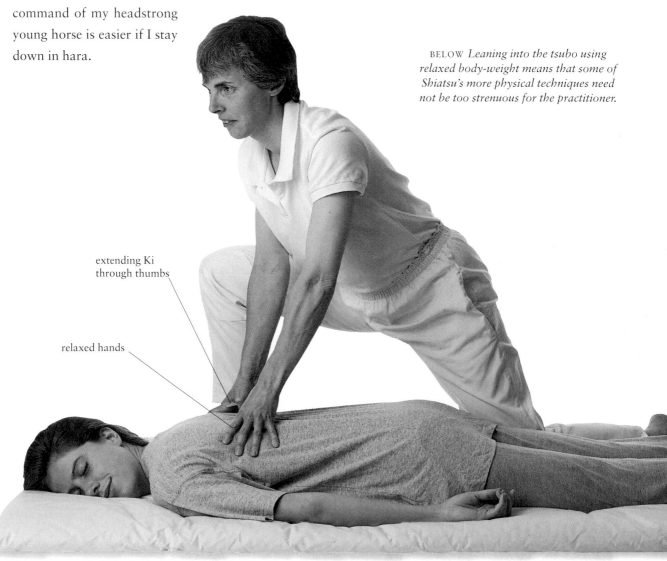

BELOW *Leaning into the tsubo using relaxed body-weight means that some of Shiatsu's more physical techniques need not be too strenuous for the practitioner.*

extending Ki
through thumbs

relaxed hands

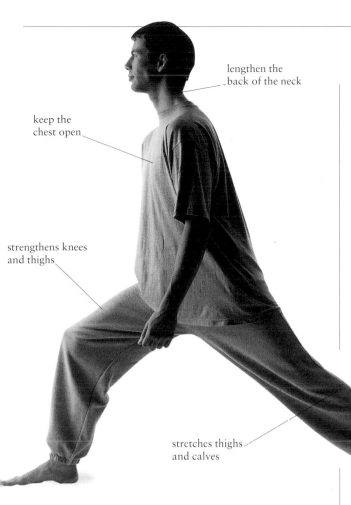

lengthen the back of the neck

keep the chest open

strengthens knees and thighs

stretches thighs and calves

ABOVE *Stretching the inner thighs develops the practitioner's body flexibility.*

EXERCISE FOR BODY FLEXIBILITY

Exercises to help you move flexibly from hara while on the floor are

◎ Stretching into a lunge position keeping your body upright – this position is used often in Shiatsu (see p. 109)

◎ Inner thigh stretching by standing with feet wide apart and allowing the body to sink down until the thighs are parallel with the floor (see above).

FINGER- AND WRIST-SUPPLING EXERCISES

People often comment on how strong my fingers and thumbs must be to apply sustained pressure. Actually, it is more to do with flexibility than strength, linked with extending Ki consciously from hara, through my hands. You may find the following finger- and wrist-suppling exercises useful.

◎ Starting with the little finger, stretch each finger in turn backward, forward, and to both sides as far as it will go. With the thumb, make sure you go backward sufficiently so that the muscle on the mound at the base of the thumb is well stretched.

◎ Bend the hand backward and forward from the wrist.

◎ With your palm facing you, grasp your hand and take the thumb away from you, creating a twist on the wrist. (Don't go too far – this is a wrist lock in aikido and can be painful.) Then return to center and work the other way with the little finger going away from you.

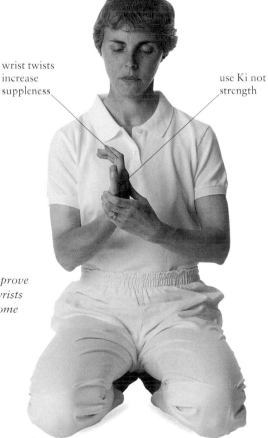

wrist twists increase suppleness

use Ki not strength

RIGHT *You can improve the power of the wrists and fingers with some simple exercises.*

When Not to Give Shiatsu

Before you start your session, there are a few general cautions that you should observe. You should not give Shiatsu in cases of fever, infectious or contagious illnesses, or on the site of burns, open sores, broken bones, or varicose veins. In the hands of an experienced practitioner, Shiatsu can be used for a wide range of health problems, but as a beginner you should not tackle any serious or acute complaint, especially cancer, heart disease, or any potentially life-threatening condition.

It is also unwise for a beginner to work on a woman during the first three months of pregnancy, and at all times during pregnancy the points SP6, LI4, and GB21 and heavy pressure below the knee should be avoided, because these points may initiate labor or cause a miscarriage. In general, work gently around any sites of pain, such as tight or pulled muscles, tendons or tenderness at joints, and if you are in doubt as to whether this basic relaxing treatment is appropriate, then take advice from an experienced practitioner.

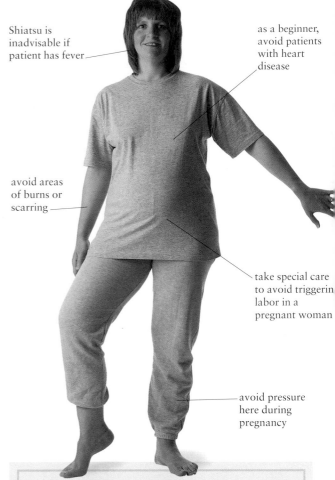

Shiatsu is inadvisable if patient has fever

as a beginner, avoid patients with heart disease

avoid areas of burns or scarring

take special care to avoid triggering labor in a pregnant woman

avoid pressure here during pregnancy

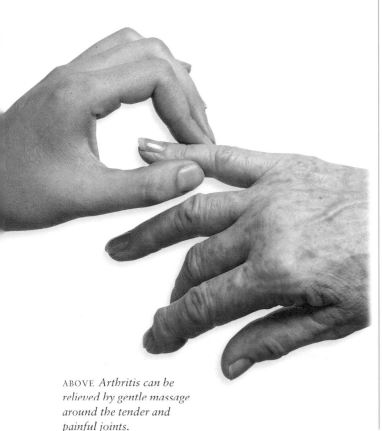

ABOVE *Arthritis can be relieved by gentle massage around the tender and painful joints.*

WHEN GIVING SHIATSU

Do

- ensure you are feeling balanced and positive.
- stay based in hara.
- keep posture open.
- have a wide base, feet or knees apart.
- use body weight to apply pressure.
- apply pressure when breathing out.
- enjoy giving Shiatsu.

Don't

- give Shiatsu when you are feeling tired, ill, or upset.
- collapse your hara.
- hunch your shoulders.
- keep feet or knees together.
- use muscular strength.
- hold your breath.
- worry about getting it "wrong."

Setting the Scene

THE ROOM SETTING

Now we are ready to begin. The room you are in is light, airy, and, above all, comfortably warm – your partner will tend to cool down as his or her metabolism slows, so warmth is important. It is good to have a blanket handy to cover hands or feet, especially if your partner has drifted off to sleep at the end of the session. A pillow is also useful to pad up knees or to put under the patient's chest when lying face downward, to ensure complete relaxation. Remember, relaxation is one of the prime benefits of Shiatsu, so your partner should be able to lie comfortably throughout the session. You may want to put on some relaxing music and perhaps burn some aromatic essential oils to enhance the peaceful atmosphere, and of course take steps to prevent interruptions from telephones, children, animals, or anything else. This is your partner's quiet time, and everything must be done to allow him or her to concentrate on that fact.

WHAT TO WEAR

It is best for both of you to wear loose cotton clothing – a sweatsuit is ideal, because it is warm and allows your partner to stretch into the various positions used in the session. Socks can be worn on the feet if they tend to get cold, but not pantyhose – it is difficult to stimulate individual toes through nylon. From your point of view, clothing that allows you to stretch and move around is essential. I find that I get quite hot as I work, and a sweatshirt is easy to slip off without losing the continuity of the session.

A FIRM SURFACE

If you have a Japanese futon, that is the ideal surface for giving Shiatsu, but a couple of blankets folded on a carpet is just as comfortable and supportive. Don't give Shiatsu to someone lying on a bed. The effect of the pressures you apply will be lost in the springs, and what is more, you will probably end up with a sore back from stooping over.

BELOW *A treatment room should be warm, airy, and restful, providing an atmosphere of calm from the start.*

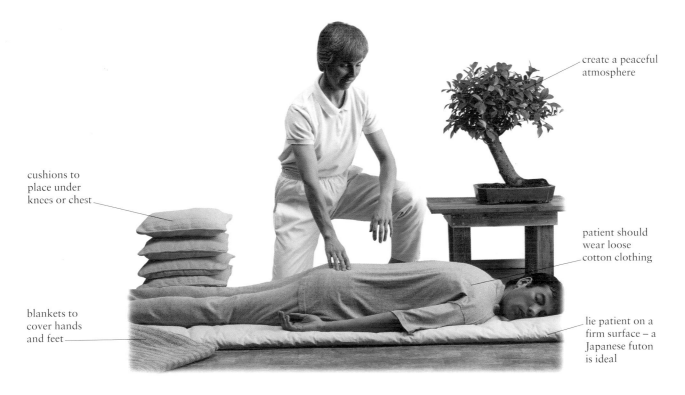

cushions to place under knees or chest

blankets to cover hands and feet

create a peaceful atmosphere

patient should wear loose cotton clothing

lie patient on a firm surface – a Japanese futon is ideal

Attitude

Your attitude in giving Shiatsu is of paramount importance, since you are using your own body and its Ki in order to help another person. This is, in fact, the essence of the spiritual development aspect of Shiatsu – being clear and balanced so as to be most effective. Calmness and concentration are the key words. You should be in a good mood, not angry, upset, preoccupied, or overtired. Try to clear away any of these negative feelings by breathing deeply into your hara and letting go all negativity as you breathe out. The human mind being what it is, unwanted thoughts like "What am I going to have for dinner?", "I must remember to phone Aunt Mary," and "Am I doing this right?" are bound to pop into your head. Just let them flow through your mind and out again; bring your concentration back to your hands and your partner – just like in meditation.

BREATHING AND CENTERING IN HARA

Breathing and centering in hara are two other important aspects that we spoke of earlier.

◎ As you sit down beside your partner, take a deep breath and let it fill up not just your lungs but the whole of your abdomen, right down to the *tanden* (the center of the hara, which is three fingers'-width below your navel).

◎ Relax and breathe right out. This recycles your own Ki and is a good technique to use at the start and finish of a session.

During the treatment, you can breathe into hara and out through your hands; this has the effect of recycling your Ki so that you avoid that unpleasant sensation of being "drained" by giving out too

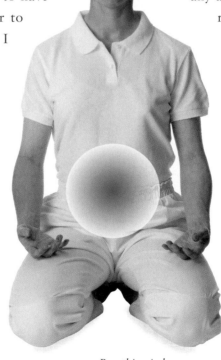

ABOVE *Breathing in hara before the session helps the practitioner let go of tension and center herself.*

much. Occasionally, too, you may come across other unwanted feelings, such as heaviness, picking up your partner's negative energy, or even getting a headache. Here again, the use of breath and also visualization can come into their own.

◎ Take a couple of deep breaths into hara to replenish your store of Ki.

◎ If your hands are feeling heavy, give them a shake, and be sure to breathe out while applying pressure, because this helps to ensure that Ki flows from you to your partner, not the other way around, which can be emotionally and physically draining for an inexperienced practitioner.

At the end of a session I always make a point of washing my hands under cold running water and breathing out a couple of times, completely emptying the lungs. This little ritual has the effect of mentally finishing off the treatment, so that I am no longer carrying the energy of that particular person around with me. The mind is a wonderfully powerful tool and can be used in instances like this to make sure that you as well as your receiver feel fulfilled and renewed at the end of the session.

When you apply pressure, keep your awareness in your hara at all times and lean into the tsubo using relaxed body-weight. This sort of pressure is much less tiring to give and much more comfortable to receive – in fact, you will probably be surprised how hard you can lean on someone when you are centered in hara and still make it pleasant. Being grounded in hara also makes you more sensitive to your partner's Ki, and you will find it much easier to tune in and give the right quantity and quality of pressure.

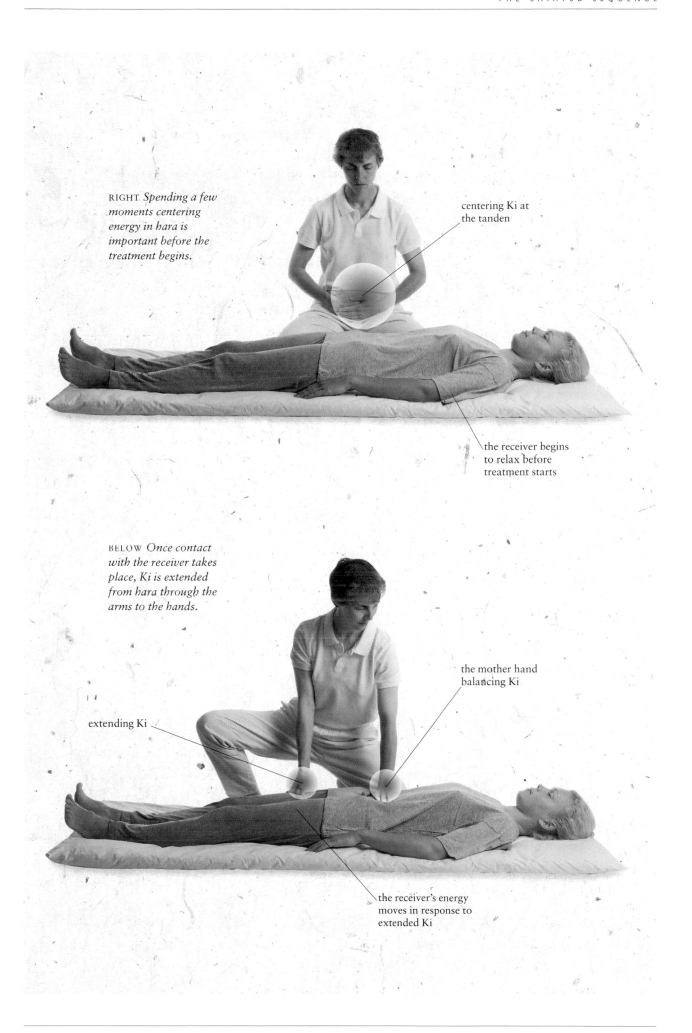

RIGHT. *Spending a few moments centering energy in hara is important before the treatment begins.*

centering Ki at the tanden

the receiver begins to relax before treatment starts

BELOW *Once contact with the receiver takes place, Ki is extended from hara through the arms to the hands.*

the mother hand balancing Ki

extending Ki

the receiver's energy moves in response to extended Ki

Pressure

Shiatsu uses the hands, thumbs, elbows, knees, and feet to apply pressure to points on the meridians. The most basic of techniques is using the thumb, the palm, or the heel of the hand straight into the body at 90 degrees (what is known in the trade as "perpendicular pressure"). We also generally work with two hands on the body; a "mother hand," which stays still, often resting on the hara or the sacrum, and a "working hand," which is the only one to apply active pressure. It is very supportive for your partner if you have two hands on at all times, helping him or her to connect up different parts of the body and increase the awareness of Self.

CONNECTING WITH KI

The pressure should be deep enough to connect with the Ki in the meridian or tsubo you are working on. If you stimulate too hard, you will hurt your partners, causing them to tighten up in order to protect

WORKING TECHNIQUES

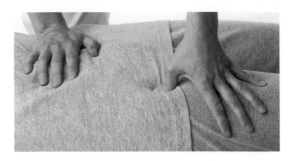

ABOVE *The "mother hand" left remains still while the thumb of the "working hand" applies very specific downward pressure.*

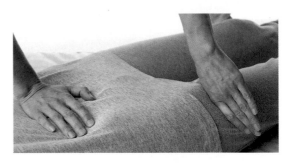

ABOVE *Working quickly over the surface with the flat of the hand relieves surface tension.*

BELOW *On heavily built people, the elbows or knees can apply stronger pressure than the hands.*

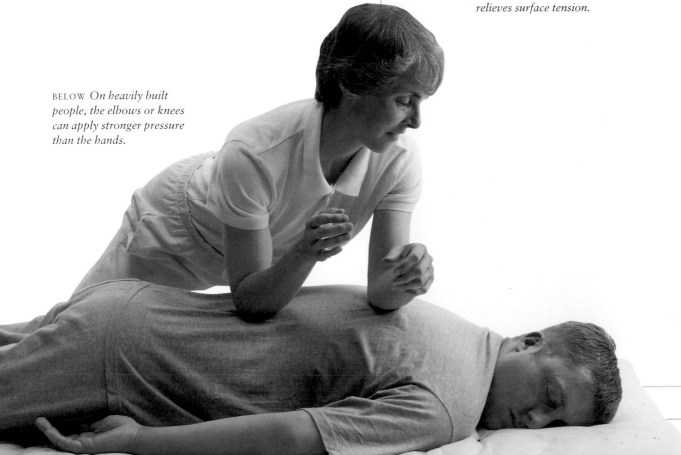

themselves. If your pressure is not sufficiently deep it will feel unsatisfactory to your partners because you won't have connected with the energy. As you concentrate and listen to your hands you will, with practice, start to tune into your partner's energy intuitively; you will then become sensitive to the degree of pressure needed.

The sensation of connecting with Ki is often accompanied by a sort of "good pain" for them, while you may feel it as a subtle change of feeling under your thumb. Don't worry if you don't feel this at first – it takes time to develop sensitivity to Ki, not to mention the confidence to know when you have connected. If you think you are feeling Ki, then you probably are! Until you are sure, the best way is to apply pressure on each point for the count of five seconds before moving on to the next point. This gives your thumb or fingers a chance to tune into the Ki of that tsubo, even though your conscious mind is not aware of connecting with Ki.

OTHER USEFUL TECHNIQUES

As well as the classic straight pressure, there are other techniques for loosening up tight muscles.
◎ Rubbing quickly over the surface with the flat of your hand is good for cold and superficial tightness.
◎ Kneading with thumbs, knuckles, or the bony part of the heel of your hand is a good way to start softening up chronically stiff muscles (especially those in the shoulder, upper back, buttock, and thigh).
◎ Having loosened up, you can then work more deeply with thumb or elbow pressure.

We always work from general techniques, palming, kneading, rotating, to more specific ones, such as holding points with thumb, elbow, or knees.

THE DIRECTION OF WORKING

Different Shiatsu techniques may work the meridians in different directions. In Zen Shiatsu, we normally work from the hara outward to the extremities, regardless of the Yin or Yang direction of flow. In practice, it is found that this is a simpler and more effective way of working, and is one we shall follow in the Basic Sequence.

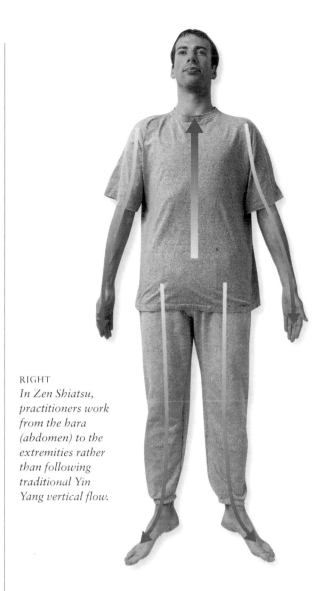

RIGHT
In Zen Shiatsu, practitioners work from the hara (abdomen) to the extremities rather than following traditional Yin Yang vertical flow.

REACTIONS TO TREATMENT

Although it is unlikely after a general Shiatsu session such as we are going to learn here, it sometimes happens that your partner may have what we term a "healing reaction" after the treatment. This may take the form of a headache, feeling tired or depressed, or possibly having flu-like symptoms that last for about 24 hours. Advise the person to drink plenty of spring water and rest to help clear the toxins that have been released, and not to worry unduly. This is the body's way of cleansing itself and is part of the healing process. If you are at all worried about reactions, please contact an experienced Shiatsu practitioner or teacher. Addresses for national associations are to be found on page 190.

② The Basic Shiatsu Sequence

The Basic Sequence that follows is a framework that will lay the foundations for your knowledge of Shiatsu, no matter at which level you wish to practice. It is a form similar to the one I teach my beginner students and is designed to stimulate all the traditional meridians to promote relaxation. Being a fairly general treatment, it is appropriate for most people, but because all the meridians and body areas are incorporated, it gives you the scope to be more specific with particular conditions and health problems in the future when you have become more sensitive and confident.

Once you have mastered the sequence to the extent that you can go through it without having to refer to the book, you will be ready to delve into the more advanced realms of hara diagnosis, tailoring your treatments to suit the condition of your receiver. Learning to do two-handed diagnosis really requires the presence of an experienced teacher to lead you through the steps and to help you interpret what you are feeling. However, the simplified form of one-handed palpation described on pages 136 and 137 can be quite accurate and, used in conjunction with the tables of meridian functions and associations, can enable you to pinpoint the appropriate meridian to work for particular imbalances.

When working through the Basic Sequence, always remember to be relaxed and comfortable – that way, your receiver will feel comfortable, too. Be aware of moving from your hara and being in touch with your breathing, both of which will help you to be more centered as well as more sensitive in your quality of touch.

Each step in the sequence should be repeated two or three times to allow the receiver to relax into each technique. Each point or pressure with palms should be held from three to five seconds.

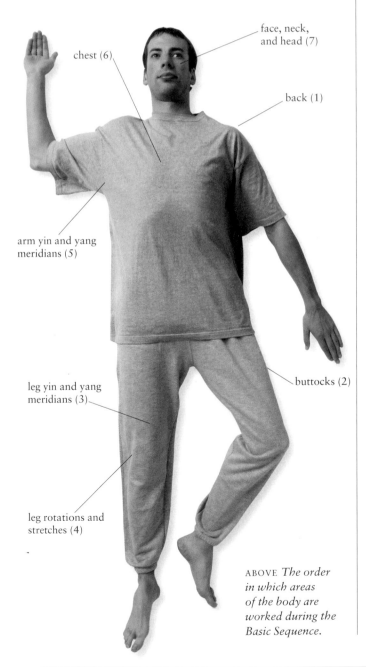

chest (6)

face, neck, and head (7)

back (1)

arm yin and yang meridians (5)

leg yin and yang meridians (3)

buttocks (2)

leg rotations and stretches (4)

ABOVE *The order in which areas of the body are worked during the Basic Sequence.*

THE BACK

The back is the part of the body in which almost everyone holds a certain amount of tension. All parts of the back are covered by layers of muscles, and in the upper back and shoulders the trapezius muscle is particularly prone to tightness. In working the thoracic area, that is, the upper back as far as the end of the ribcage, you can work relatively strongly, since the ribs protect the internal organs. However, in the lumbar area, between the ribs and the hip bones, you must be more careful since this is usually more sensitive and weaker. The sacrum, the bony triangle at the base of the spine, is an area where people often like medium, supportive pressure: it can be sensitive in women and those with chronic back problems.

THE BASIC SEQUENCE IN SUMMARY

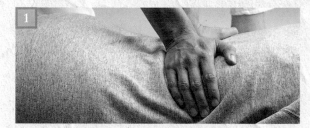

The lower back is worked mainly by using firm pressure with the palm and heel of the hand.

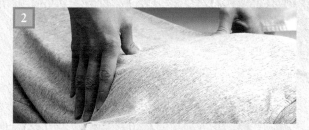

Tension between the shoulder blades is relieved by thumbing the Bladder meridian.

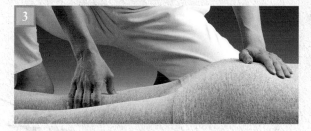

Buttocks and thighs are thumbed or palmed, with the mother hand providing light support on the sacrum.

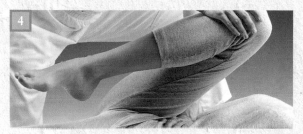

Leg stretches, such as stretching each knee to the opposite shoulder, activate supplementary meridians.

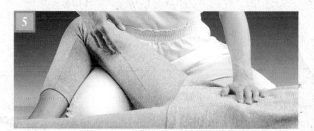

Accessing the Liver meridian is achieved by working on the inner thigh.

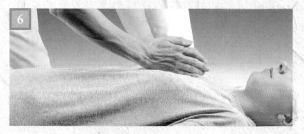

The chest has to be worked carefully, usually with the side of the hands.

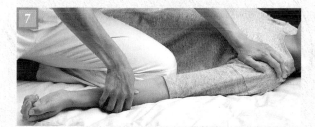

The arm is held straight and palmed, then thumbed, along the Heart Governor meridian.

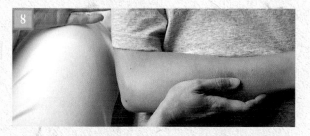

Outstretched fingertips are used to stimulate the Triple Heater meridian.

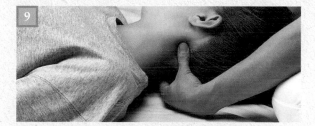

The fingers are used to stimulate GB20, situated between the two large neck muscles.

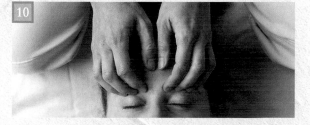

Gentle facial stimulation completes the sequences, leaving the receiver deeply relaxed.

The Back

When working the back, always work from the shoulders downward to the sacrum. If you keep your arms nearly straight you will be less inclined to use muscle power. Ask your receiver to lie face down with arms by his or her sides. Your receiver may move his or her head from side to side to prevent stiffness, and, if necessary, pad under the chest with a pillow if the neck is uncomfortable. Don't support the head with a pillow, since this is likely to put excess strain on the neck.

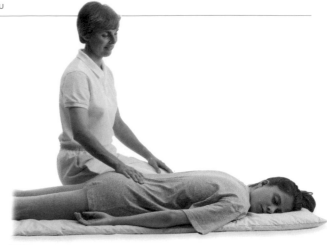

1 *"Make friends" by sitting beside your receiver in seiza, with your hand on the sacrum. Take a couple of deep breaths down into hara and be aware of warmth from your hand extending down into the sacrum.*

MERIDIANS

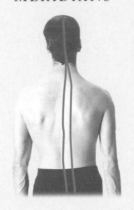

The Bladder (BL) meridian is the longest in the body, arising at the inner corners of the eye and running over the head and neck to the top of the back. Two pairs of BL lines run down the back: the inner pair lie 1.5 cun (thumbs' width) from the spine, the outer pair 3 cun from the spine. The BL pathway continues down the back of the leg to the little toe. The BL meridian governs the urinary system, the bones (particularly the spinal column), and the autonomic nervous system. Of special interest are the Yu points (see page 76), which are situated on the inner BL line in the back. Points parallel to the Yu points on the outer BL line are used to treat the emotional aspect of the same organ.

RIGHT *Before beginning the sequence, prepare yourself by sitting in seiza (see p. 44) and centering in the hara.*

take deep breaths in preparation

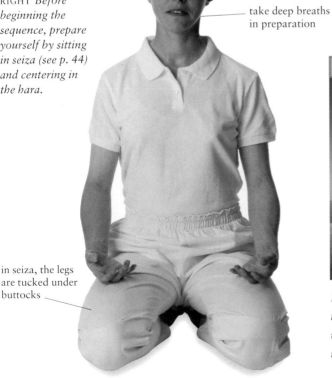

in seiza, the legs are tucked under buttocks

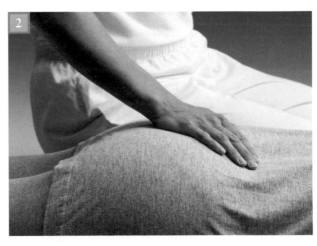

Rock the sacrum from side to side, keeping your hand on the same area (this is a "rock," not a "rub"). Allow the movement to swing so that the receiver's whole body is moving right down to the toes.

3 *Come up onto one knee into a lunge position. Leave your mother hand on the sacrum. With your working hand, lean on your palm to one side of the spine, and continue down to the sacrum. Repeat on the other side.*

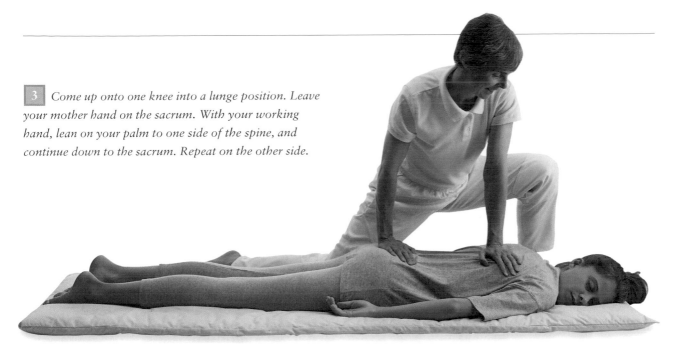

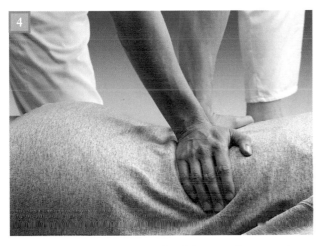

Place both hands on either side of the spine between the shoulder blades. Lean down onto the heels of your hands as you breathe out. Continue down the spine to the sacrum, holding each pressure for 3 to 5 seconds.

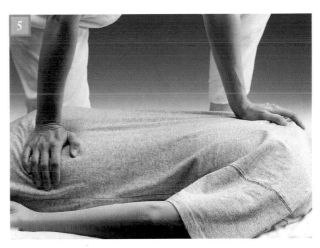

Place one hand on one buttock and the other on the opposite side of the back, between the spine and the shoulder blade. Lean in between your hands to create a diagonal stretch. Reverse and repeat.

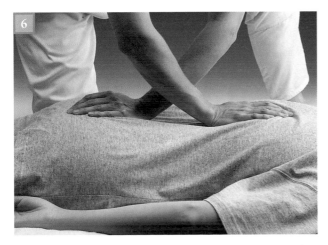

Place the heel of one hand at the top of the sacrum, and place the other at the first lumbar vertebra (just above the small of the back) with wrists crossing. Push your hands away from each other to make a lumbar stretch.

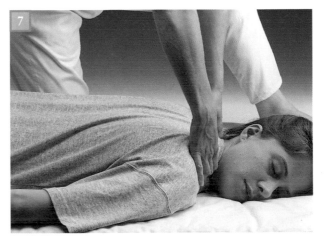

Take the shoulder muscles, one in each hand, and make kneading movements with thumbs and fingers to loosen them up. You are working on the top of the trapezius muscle, which often holds a lot of tension.

The Upper Back and Shoulders

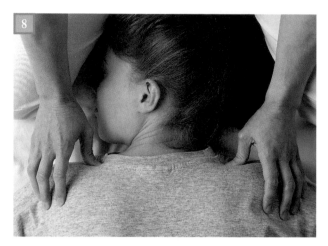

Move to a kneeling position above the head. Thumb along the top of the trapezius muscle from the neck to the shoulder joint. The direction of pressure is toward the receiver's toes. If your receiver is pregnant, do not press GB21 in the middle of this line; it may initiate labor.

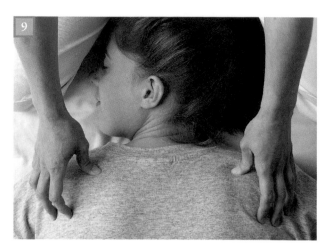

Feel for the ridge of bone on the shoulder blade. Thumb from the center outward along the muscle on the upper side of this ridge.

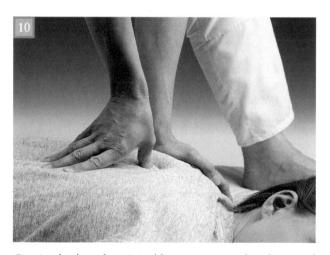

Coming back to the original lunge position, thumb around the inner border of the shoulder blade from top to point.

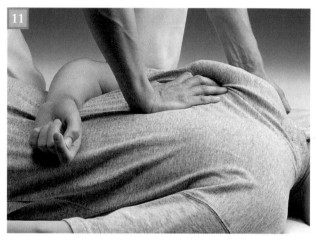

Place your receiver's arm across the back, supporting the receiver's elbow with your ankle. Place your fingers to the side of the shoulder blade, and leaning back, lift the shoulder with your other hand so that the shoulder blade rolls over your fingertips. Working from the point of the shoulder blade upward makes this technique easier.

12 Starting level with the top of the shoulder blades, place your thumbs one and a half cun out from the spine on both sides, and breathing out from hara, lean down onto your thumbs with arms nearly straight. Work the Yu points on the Bladder meridian. Slide your thumbs down an inch and lean in again. Continue down to the sacrum, where your thumbs will tend to come closer together. Remember, it is important to move from hara when working on the Yu points. Repeat the whole line of Yu points, from shoulder blades to the tip of the sacrum, three times.

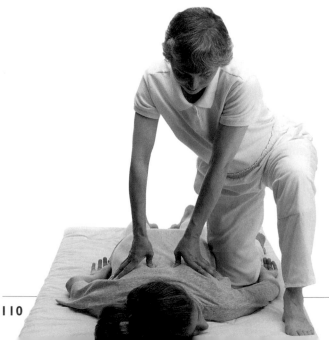

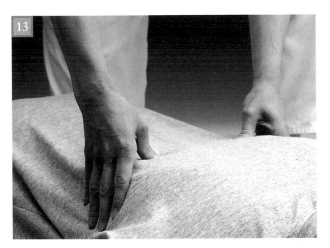

Go back up to the top of the back, and this time, thumb two lines parallel to the spine three thumbs' width from the midline. This is the second line of the Bladder meridian, which extends down over the buttock area.

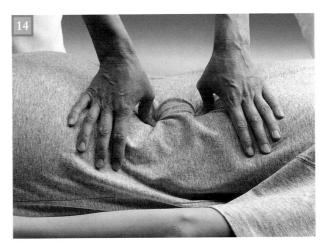

Advanced technique: Having worked both inner and outer branches of the BL meridian, if there is particular tension on one side of the back you can work just that affected portion, using two thumbs on the same side of the spine.

CASE HISTORY
Mr. B., male, 50 years

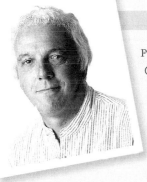

PRESENTING SYMPTOMS: Chronic muscular tension in the neck, shoulders, and upper back, resulting in crushing headaches at the back and side of the head. Stress.

MEDICAL HISTORY: In his own words, he has always been "disgustingly healthy!"

BACKGROUND: Very high-stress, high-profile job in showbusiness. Alternating periods of sitting over a computer (he acknowledged his posture was not as good as it used to be), with extreme activity when performing in public.

DIAGNOSIS: Over a series of treatments, a pattern appeared of either TH or ST kyo and GB or BL jitsu.

TREATMENT: All four of these Yang meridians run in the head and neck, so it was very easy to work on his muscular tension and head pain by accessing these meridians. Obviously, each had to be worked differently according to its energetic status, with Bladder and Gall Bladder in the neck, shoulders, and upper back being stimulated extensively.

On the first treatment he was recovering from a headache. When he traced the location of the pain pattern, it was very clearly due to a disturbance in the Gall Bladder meridian, since it followed the course of the meridian exactly. Initially, I spent a lot of time loosening up his shoulders by using steps 7 to 9, because these techniques move stuck energy in the trapezius muscle. This prepared him for step 11, working under the shoulder blade, and he felt quite a bit of relief in the shoulders and neck afterward. Toward the end of the session we also worked on the Gall Bladder meridian in the neck in supine position (steps 50 and 51 on pp.130 and 131) as well as steps 52 and 53 (pp.132 and 133) which de-activate tightness in the sternocleidomastoid muscle (SCM). Because both the trapezius and the SCM attach into the head, tightness in them can cause head pain by the action of trigger points (see page 91). This pattern of treatment was repeated in subsequent sessions, and by the third session, he reported that he had suffered from no headaches between our meetings.

The Buttocks

Everyone tends to hold a lot of tension in their buttocks, and some also hold stagnation here in the form of fat. The muscles in the buttock area are concerned basically with moving the thigh and stabilizing the pelvis. Because they are postural muscles, they tend to become overtense under stress.

WORKING THE BUTTOCKS

The piriformis muscle runs from the inside of the sacrum to the top of the femur and rotates the leg outward. This muscle is particularly prone to tightness, which can often affect the sciatic nerve, resulting in sciatic pain radiating as far down as the knee, as well as pain in the lower back and buttock area. Deep, slow, holding pressure can be very effective in relieving tightness here.

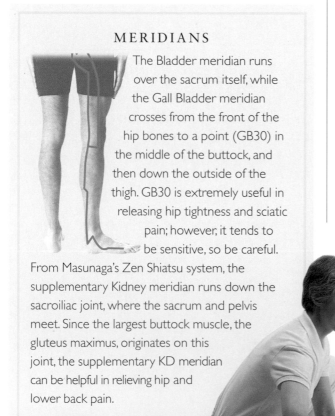

MERIDIANS

The Bladder meridian runs over the sacrum itself, while the Gall Bladder meridian crosses from the front of the hip bones to a point (GB30) in the middle of the buttock, and then down the outside of the thigh. GB30 is extremely useful in releasing hip tightness and sciatic pain; however, it tends to be sensitive, so be careful. From Masunaga's Zen Shiatsu system, the supplementary Kidney meridian runs down the sacroiliac joint, where the sacrum and pelvis meet. Since the largest buttock muscle, the gluteus maximus, originates on this joint, the supplementary KD meridian can be helpful in relieving hip and lower back pain.

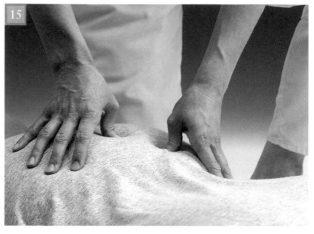

Thumb down the sacroiliac joint from the crest of the hip bone to the coccyx. Remember to keep your pressure at 90 degrees and allow your thumbs to taper in as you follow the triangular shape of the sacrum.

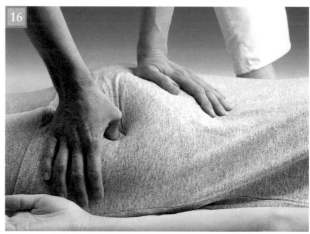

Find the sensitive point in the center of the buttock. This is GB30, located two thirds of the way down a line from the coccyx to the top of the femur (thigh bone). Press three times with your thumb. This may feel tender to the receiver.

17 *Place the heels of both hands into the hollows at the sides of the buttocks and, alternating pressure between one hand and the other, make large circular movements forward, keeping your hand on the same piece of flesh rather than rubbing.*

CASE HISTORY
Mr. L., male, 35 years

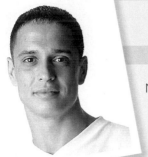

Mr L. arrived for "emergency" treatment, having telephoned to say he needed Shiatsu urgently for severe back pain. The urgency of the situation became clear to me when Mr L. explained that he was a classical dancer by profession and was supposed to lead some workshops with a small dance company, culminating in performances in a week's time. Considering his posture and his very careful movement while getting in and out of a chair, I was doubtful whether he would be fit to do the sort of strenuous workout he described as normal for these performances; however, we agreed to "see what we could do."

PRESENTING SYMPTOMS: The pain was principally on the left side and fluctuated from above the sacrum to the coccyx. The previous day he had been doing extensive floor exercises and he felt this had aggravated an old injury. When asked for details of this, it transpired that he had broken the head of his femur (the very top part of the thigh bone, close to the ball-and-socket joint) two years previously and had subsequently lost a lot of outward rotation in the leg. This latter loss of movement is quite serious for a classical dancer, as turnout is important in ballet. He felt that possibly he compensated for this in other movements and reported a certain amount of play on the knee joint as well as pain behind the knee.

TREATMENT: In the first session I concentrated on the Bladder meridian, doing extensive work on the lumbar points, especially the Kidney and Large Intestine Yu points (step 12). On working down the Bladder points in the sacrum and on the supplementary Kidney at the edge of the sacrum (step 15), I found that he was very sensitive on the left side and the muscles in the buttocks on the left looked distinctly more taut. Having spent some time gently loosening these up with long slow pressure, I was then able to do the buttock circling technique described in step 17. This was followed with specific work on the piriformis muscle, which runs deep under gluteus maximus, and

pressure on BL36 (in the middle of the crease just below the buttock) and BL57 (directly below the end of the gastrocnemius, or calf muscle), both of which are traditional points for back pain relief (step 18).

At the second session Mr. L felt better, with a slight pain across the sacrum and his left side stiffer than the right. His posture was more upright and generally he looked more comfortable, though not with the kind of fluid movement one would expect from a dancer. The Kidney was showing more energy today, but the Triple Heater was somewhat down. He remarked that his intestines had been upset the previous week after he had been taking alcohol and drugs. I felt that his Lower Heater was out of balance, and included some work on the hara. Most of the session followed the same format as previously: trying to relieve the tightness in the left buttock and working the lumbar points of the Bladder meridian. There was less generalized tightness and I was able to feel that there was a knot of tense muscle between the fourth and fifth lumbar vertebrae. As we worked this began to relax, the left side being more reactive. Since he was generally looser, I could get his legs into the stretch position for the Gall Bladder (see step 19), which made it easier to get deeper into the gluteal muscles, especially GB30, an excellent point for sciatic and leg pain.

By the third session five days later, he was reporting only localized pain at the left sacroiliac joint. The other spasms and aches had gone, so although we worked extensively on the back I was also able to address a Fire imbalance involving his Heart meridian, which was also significant in the next treatment, which took place four days later, and although he felt somewhat stiff on the left, his acute pain had gone.

Our last treatment was two days later on the first day of his performance. By now his back was sufficiently strong and comfortable that he reported he had been able to do some lifting. When I asked in consternation if that was really necessary, he explained that it was — he was lifting people during the ballet! I concluded from this that the treatment had sorted out his problem as far as he was concerned!

Leg Yang Meridians

The leg Yang meridians, which are accessible to the practitioner when the receiver is in this pı position, are the Bladder and Gall Bla meridians. The Bladder meridian r down the back of the leg and is treate with the leg straight, while the Gal Bladder runs on the outside of the leg and is treated with the leg bent up. There are several useful points for treating back pain on the BL meridian in the leg: BL36 just below the buttock, BL40 in the center of the back of the knee, BL56 in the center of the calf muscle, and BL57 just below the calf.

WORKING LEG YANG MERIDIANS

You should always be aware that these tsubo (see p. 26) may be quite tender. The Gall Bladder meridian is also often sensitive, possibly owing to the fact that one of its functions is to assist in the digestion of fats, and the Western diet tends to be overrich in oils and fat. Working the Gall Bladder can be particularly useful for general stiffness. (The third of the Yang meridians, the Stomach, will be dealt with in the supine position.)

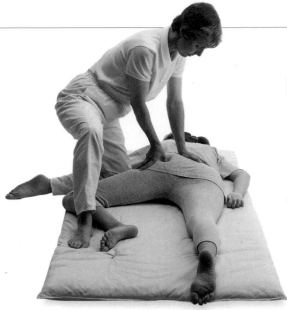

19 *Bend the foot up toward the buttock, then slide the knee outward to expose the side of the leg. Palm, then thumb the GB meridian, ending at the fourth toe.*

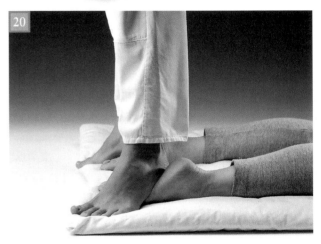

Straighten the leg carefully and move to the feet. Stand up and place the soles of your feet on the receiver's, keeping your toes on the floor for balance. Now repeat steps 18 and 19 on the other leg. Then ask your receiver to roll over onto his or her back.

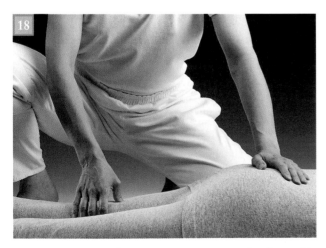

Keeping your mother hand on the sacrum, palm down the BL meridian in the back of the leg. Then thumb the same line, paying attention to the points mentioned above. Squeeze the Achilles tendon and down to the little toe.

MERIDIAN

The Gall Bladder meridian travels the whole length of the outside of the body, and one of its features is that it has a zigzag pathway that sometimes makes it difficult to follow. However, the part of GB that is being worked here is easy in that it runs from GB30 in the buttock right down the outside of the thigh and lower leg to the fourth toe. The Gall Bladder meridian is responsible for the secretion of bile, smooth movement of the joints, and, on a psychological level, decision-making.

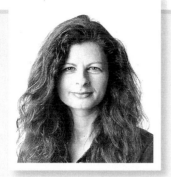

CASE HISTORY
Mrs. H., female, 40 years

PRESENTING SYMPTOMS: Mrs. H. was receiving ongoing treatment for premenstrual syndrome and migraines. On two occasions she developed acute lower back pain.

MEDICAL HISTORY: Severe depression in the week leading up to her period, coupled with migraines and intestinal upset.

DIAGNOSIS: On both occasions (several months apart), the diagnosis was KD kyo, LI jitsu. This denotes a combination of coldness and weakness in the upper lumbar area and tight holding at the lower lumbar and buttocks.

TREATMENT: On both occasions we spent considerable time working on the immediate problem, with the ongoing imbalance going "onto the back burner." She had been practicing some exercises and had overstretched, resulting in the deep muscles on one side of the spine going into spasm. Her posture was very protective and curled to one side, and she was afraid she had "put her back out." I could assure her that all the bones were in place, but that the deep muscles on one side of the spinal column had seized up in response to the unaccustomed stretch.

Since there was also an emotional component to her imbalance, I worked gently on the upper back part of the Bladder meridian, before palming in the lumbar area (steps 3 and 4). With gentle thumb pressure on Ahshi points in the region of pain, the muscles began to relax (step 14). A balancing stretch, with her lying on her back, helped to ease out the muscles even further (step 21), and she went away feeling much less sore. Subsequent treatments removed the pain altogether.

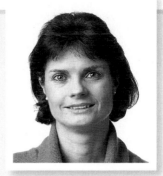

CASE HISTORY
Ms. J., female, 30 years

PRESENTING SYMPTOMS: Chronic lower back pain focused in the coccyx.

MEDICAL HISTORY: Hysterectomy one year ago, now on HRT and experiencing many menopausal symptoms as well as PMS. Gaining weight since the operation, and also has IBS (Irritable Bowel Syndrome) dating from then.

BACKGROUND: Young mother with two lively daughters, aged 10 and 12. Cheerful disposition, works parttime in a caring environment, finds her pain and lack of mobility depressing.

DIAGNOSIS: TH kyo, BL jitsu.

TREATMENT: At her first treatment, in addition to back pain, Ms. J. was suffering acutely from a toothache. On examination it was obvious that her sacroiliac joint was out of place on the right. Having first adjusted that, I then worked on the Bladder meridian, with Ms. J. in a prone position, lying face downward. However, this felt uncomfortable to her, so I used side position (see specialist techniques for back pain on page 172). We spent a lot of time very gently stimulating the Bladder meridian, which despite being jitsu, or excessive, did not feel as if it could take any robust sedating work at all. Since the Bladder was involved in the diagnosis, I worked along as much of the meridian as I could. In particular, the points on Bladder in the leg (as in step 18) were very useful. I also used points in her hands and on her face to help control the tooth pain for the duration of the session (later she made an appointment with the dentist and had an abscess drained). After the treatment she was able to sit up by herself, which was a great improvement.

Leg Rotations

Leg rotations have several functions. Firstly, at this stage in the Basic Sequence they act as a complement to all the work that has been done on the back, by curling the back in the opposite direction and therefore making sure it remains supple. Secondly, rotating the legs, either both together or singly, is extremely useful in loosening up the lower back and the hip joints. Mobility in the hips is important for posture, for avoiding lower back pain, and keeping people active, especially in old age. Being relaxed and mobile in the pelvic area facilitates the functioning of the intestines and bladder, the reproductive organs, and it also enhances and facilitates sexual activity.

WORKING LEG ROTATIONS

When doing the following leg rotations and twists, it is important for you to be very well grounded in your hara; otherwise you may lose balance or strain to hold up your receiver's legs. Keep your feet well apart and your knees bent.

MERIDIAN

The Stomach meridian is the third leg Yang meridian, and its pathway is from the face, down the torso and along the front of the thigh and lower leg, ending at the second toe. The part of the ST that is being worked here begins at the front of the groin, running down the thigh and in the lower leg just to the outside of the tibia. Deep work in the groin and upper thigh can access the psoas muscle, often implicated in lower back pain, while ST 36 below the knee is good for general strengthening and vitality, tired and painful legs, and digestive disorders. The ST meridian governs upper digestive functions, and on a psychological level is to do with the way people nurture themselves, so can have an impact on self-esteem.

21 *Pick up your receiver's legs by holding just under the knees. Push both knees toward the chest, being sensitive to how far you go. Hold for 10 seconds and release. Repeat three times.*

CAUTION

When you straighten the legs at the end of step 23, do so by holding under the knees; never hold at the ankles, because the knee may snap open, causing serious injury.

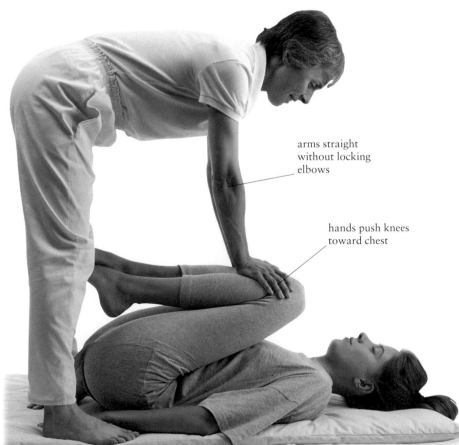

arms straight without locking elbows

hands push knees toward chest

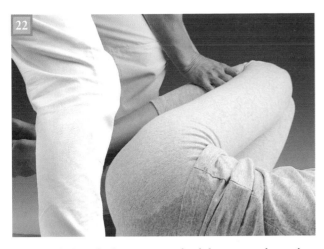

Holding below the knees, swing both legs around together in as large a circle as is comfortable for your receiver. Rotate three times in each direction.

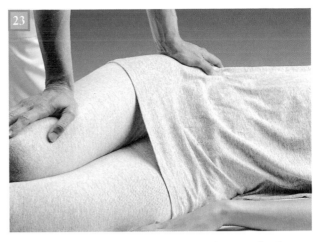

Keeping the legs bent, take both knees down to the floor on one side, hold for 10 seconds, and then take to the other side and hold. This creates a nice twist on the lower back. Straighten the legs, remembering the caution in step 21.

CAUTION

SP6 should not be used during pregnancy since heavy stimulation here can cause miscarriage in early pregnancy, or even premature labor.

24 Place the mother hand on the receiver's hara, and with the working hand, pick up the leg nearest you just below the knee, then rotate slowly three times in each direction. This is good for increasing hip mobility.

If you found the previous rotation difficult to accomplish correctly while keeping a hand on hara, you can do the same rotation holding at knee and ankle. Go as far as is comfortable for your receiver.

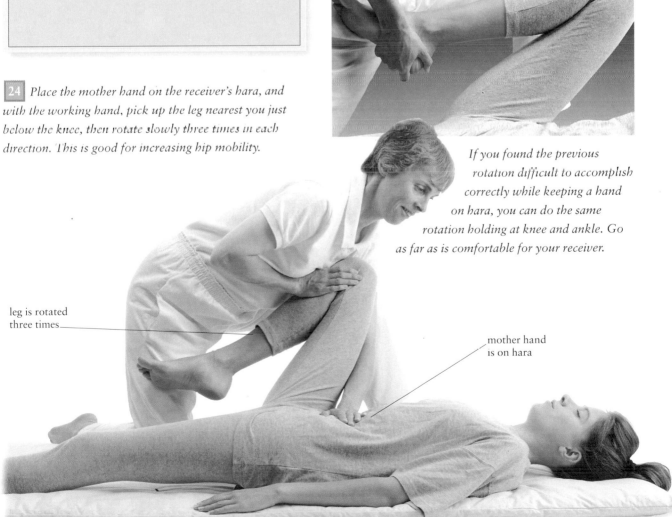

leg is rotated three times

mother hand is on hara

Leg Stretches and ST Meridian

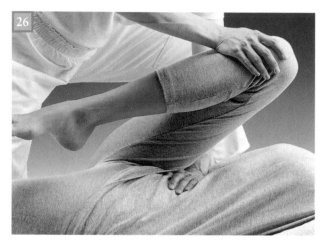

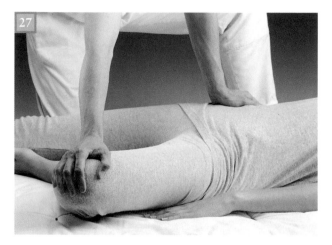

Following on from the previous rotations, stretch the knee to the opposite shoulder. This is activating the supplementary KD meridian, which runs to the outside of the hamstrings and also stretches the piriformis and other gluteal muscles in the buttocks.

Place the instep of the leg you are holding halfway up the calf and let the knee rotate outward to create a stretch on the inner thigh. Support the opposite hip bone and allow the weight of your working hand to make the stretch.

28 Advanced technique: Supporting the same side shoulder, place your receiver's foot on the opposite side of the knee. Ask the receiver to breathe out, while you push the knee away to form a strong lumbar twist.

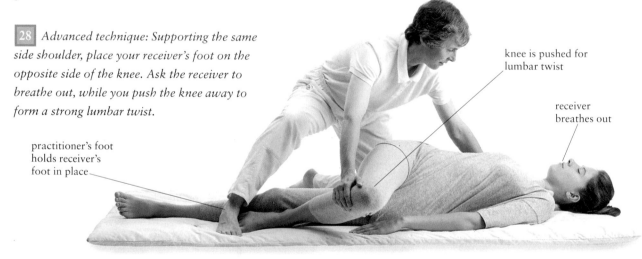

knee is pushed for lumbar twist

receiver breathes out

practitioner's foot holds receiver's foot in place

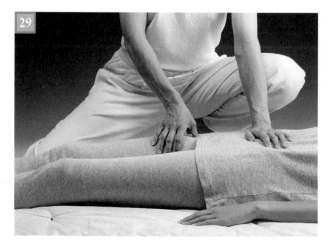

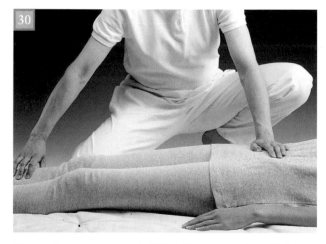

Thumb the ST meridian, starting in the groin; be careful, since this area is sensitive. Continue down the front of the thigh in line with the outside of the kneecap.

Below the knee, stimulate ST36 (four fingers' width below the knee and one thumb's width out from the tibia). Press down the lower leg, across the foot to end on the second toe.

118

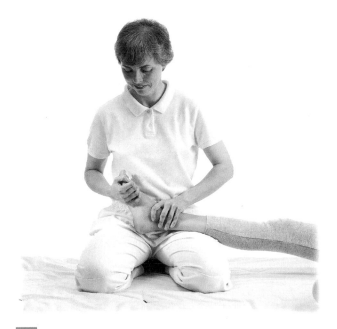

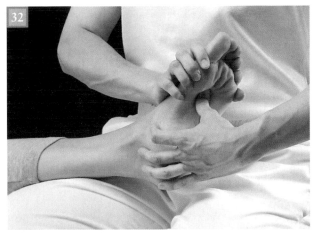

31 *Cradle the foot against your hara. Rotate the ankle in both directions, then stretch up and down. With your thumbs, work between the bones on top of the foot, from ankle to toes. Rotate each toe in turn.*

Press LV3 in the hollow behind the second joint of the big toe. With a loose fist, tap lightly all over the sole. Press KD1 in the center, just below the ball of the foot. Smooth off the foot by brushing from ankle to toes.

CASE HISTORY
Mrs. T., female, 50 years

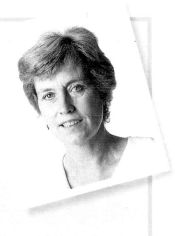

PRESENTING SYMPTOMS: Pain in lower back on walking and standing still (better for sitting in an upright chair) for 13 years. Has also had five car crashes in the last 13 years, resulting in whiplash on several occasions. Frequent heartburn.

MEDICAL HISTORY: Total hysterectomy six years ago, followed by what she terms "total body collapse," including loss of voice for nine months, hiatus hernia, throat surgery, depression.

BACKGROUND: Unhappy childhood, and unhappy marriage that she left 12 years ago. Brought up children with no support from their father. Starting to do work that she finds interesting and inspirational.

DIAGNOSIS: Ongoing pattern of ST kyo, LI jitsu.

ANALYSIS: There had been a long-term lack of nurturing in her home environment, leading to low self-esteem in the past. The hysterectomy, hiatus hernia, whiplash, and throat problems had all affected the physical area of the ST meridian. There was therefore depletion on both the emotional and physical aspects of ST.

The Large Intestine is physically in charge of eliminating waste products from the body, and on a mental or emotional level its function is to rid the Self of old, unwanted thoughts and feelings, the "old baggage" of the past that people tend to carry in their minds. On the days when she presented with LI jitsu, there was frequently some issue from the past (often relating to old relationships) that was surfacing, and was proving difficult for her to let go of.

TREATMENT: Except for working gently on the area of back pain, the most effective technique was working on the ST meridian in the groin area (step 29). Here I used slow, deep pressure, holding tender points for up to a minute. This helped to tonify a particularly weak part of the ST meridian, and also assisted in relaxing the insertion of the iliopsoas muscle (usually known as psoas for short), which is commonly shortened and tight in people with lower back pain.

Leg Yin Meridians

The Yin meridians are located on the soft inner surfaces of the leg. The inner thigh can be quite tender and work here may feel very intimate: all three Yin meridians (Spleen, Liver, and Kidney) are involved with people's reproductive and sexual life. Be sensitive to your receiver's feelings, and don't work deeply if this feels intrusive.

WORKING THE LEG YIN MERIDIANS

You may find it awkward to achieve 90-degree pressure on the thigh using your thumb, so use fingertips, side of hand, or elbows instead. Be careful with varicose veins. Three different stretch positions are used for working that ensure that each meridian is at an easily accessible angle. As you move from one meridian to the next you can do a leg rotation (as step 24) to make a smooth transition.

33 *Pick up the leg, rotate, and place the instep beside the opposite ankle, allowing the knee to fall outward and be supported on your knee. Remember to place the mother hand on hara. Using elbows on SP in the thigh can give strong, relaxed pressure through the large muscles. Below the knee use your thumb.*

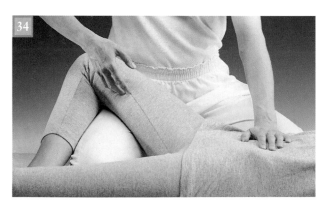

Using palms, then fingertips, access Liver in the inner thigh behind the prominent adductor muscles, with the instep placed to the opposite knee. Below the knee, thumb along the front of the tibia, diverting into SP6, and continuing to the inside of the big toe.

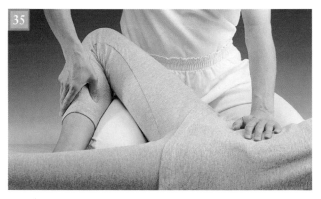

The traditional Kidney meridian is found by bending the knee even farther and working quite far around toward the back of the thigh. Then work down the calf behind the ankle to the sole of the foot.

CASE HISTORY
Miss R., female, 30 years

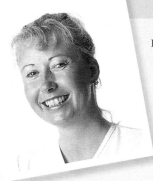

PRESENTING SYMPTOMS: Miss R. is a very athletic young woman who enjoys sports, especially cross-country running. This activity was being hampered by problems around the time of her monthly period, ranging from migraines with vomiting, and feeling weak for five to seven days around the period, to painful menstrual flow, premenstrual cravings for salty food, and a drop in her hormone levels during the immediate post-menstrual days.

MEDICAL HISTORY: She had always suffered from headaches with vomiting throughout her life, but otherwise was very healthy.

BACKGROUND: Menstrual and reproductive problems can occur in Spleen or Kidney meridians. However, Miss R.'s craving for salty food coupled with her liking for cold, wintery weather, her tendency to tire easily, and a family history of nervous system or kidney problems pointed definitely to something going on in the Water Element.

DIAGNOSIS: KD presented as kyo at all four treatments, with ST low on two occasions. Jitsu was either LI or LU.

TREATMENT: Having loosened up the upper back and shoulders and worked generally on the BL meridian to help with the headaches, at all four sessions I concentrated on the Yin meridians on the inside of the legs (steps 33 to 36), especially the Kidney meridian, which had been showing a lack of Ki flow (step 35). Kidney points around the inner ankle are particularly useful for menstrual problems, so these were worked extensively. LV3 was also used, since it is a powerful point in reducing migraines and bringing rising energy in the head back down into the body. The "meeting or three Yin streams" SP6 was not only stimulated during treatment, but also given to Miss R. as "homework" to press every day, especially before her period.

Over the course of the series of treatments, Miss R. had two periods. With both of these there was less pain, no migraines, and only a slight headache for two days, coupled with a feeling of tiredness, which passed with an hour's rest (as opposed to the usual day or two off work). She felt this to be a significant improvement on her pretreatment condition.

CAUTION

SP6 should not be used during pregnancy, since heavy stimulation here can cause miscarriage.

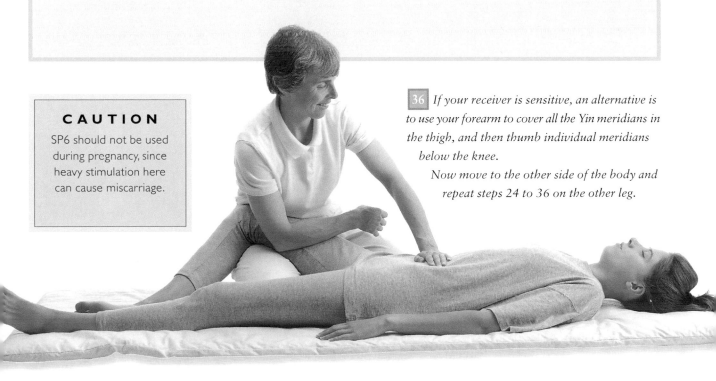

36 *If your receiver is sensitive, an alternative is to use your forearm to cover all the Yin meridians in the thigh, and then thumb individual meridians below the knee.*

Now move to the other side of the body and repeat steps 24 to 36 on the other leg.

The Hara

The hara is a sensitive and personal area that most people are not used to having touched. It may therefore take a few moments for your receiver to relax and open to you, so be patient. Working directly on the hara means you can stimulate the intestines and help them to eliminate old waste that may have been caught there, producing a buildup of toxins. The female reproductive organs are in the lower hara, and working here can help with menstrual problems as well as preventing the buildup of waste and toxins in the ovaries and uterus.

WORKING THE HARA

Always remember to work slowly and smoothly in the hara, starting any technique lightly before going deeper, and coming to an end again more gently. If your partner is a woman, ask where she is in her menstrual cycle, because hara work just before or during the period may be uncomfortable; work gently if this is the case.

MERIDIAN

Spleen, Liver, Stomach, and Kidney meridians all run in parallel lines through the hara. In addition, there is the Conception Vessel, which runs up the midline. The Conception Vessel influences Yin within the body and is noteworthy in that on it are some of the Bo points, which can be used as diagnostic points in the same manner as the Yu points on the back.

Since the Yin front of the body tends to be more sensitive than the back, many of these points can be tender, and care should be taken not to work too deeply.

By using the two general techniques described below you will automatically stimulate points on all of these meridians. Later, when you are more experienced, specific points in the hara can be added to your routine.

37 *Sit facing your partner. Place one hand over the other on your receiver's hara and slowly rock your body backward and forward, making a push-pull action, a bit like kneading dough slowly. Don't rub, but keep in touch with the same area of flesh. Work for 3 full minutes, beginning and ending gently.*

CAUTION
Be careful working over sites of past abdominal surgery as scar tissue or adhesions may be tender. Use light pressure if there is intestinal blockage.

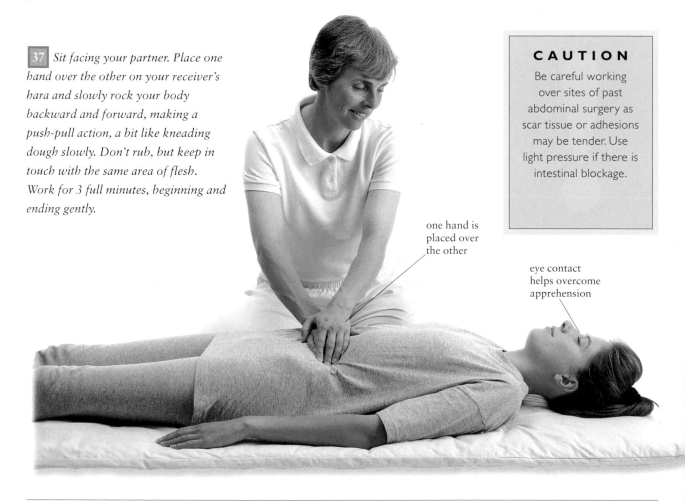

one hand is placed over the other

eye contact helps overcome apprehension

CASE HISTORY
Miss V., female, 25 years

The simplest treatments are often the most effective. This case was recounted to me by one of my graduate students, who was delighted with the success of a couple of very short treatments.

PRESENTING SYMPTOMS: The patient was a 25-year-old woman who suffered from Irritable Bowel Syndrome and was under a great deal of stress.

MEDICAL HISTORY: She had been on different types of medication for nine months, with continuing alternating diarrhea and constipation. Her life was ruled by her intestinal problems and six months previously she had had a nervous breakdown. Premenstrual syndrome was also a problem for her, with regular migraines and abdominal bloating.

BACKGROUND: Miss V.'s mother also suffered from Irritable Bowel Syndrome and was physically disabled. Stress seemed to be a major factor throughout Miss V.'s life.

TREATMENT: These were relatively short and involved mostly the "hara rocking" technique shown in step 37, and pressure on LV3 to help with the migraines. After the first session, bowel movements began to be more regular, and since the second treatment she has had two movements per day, with no bloating, constipation, or diarrhea. There was a lot of release of emotional tension at the time, resulting in Miss V. reducing her antidepressant medication intake from three tablets to one per day (this was with the consent of her family doctor). Premenstrual symptoms were much improved, with no migraines and very few headaches since her treatments. She is off all laxatives and intestinal medication.

Miss V. stated that she ceased to have worries about going out and not knowing where the next toilet might be, to the extent that she was confident enough to go away on a vacation. Her mother was adamant that the improvement stemmed from the time my graduate student used the hara rocking treatment. Miss V.'s relieved comment was that the Irritable Bowel Syndrome "no longer rules my life."

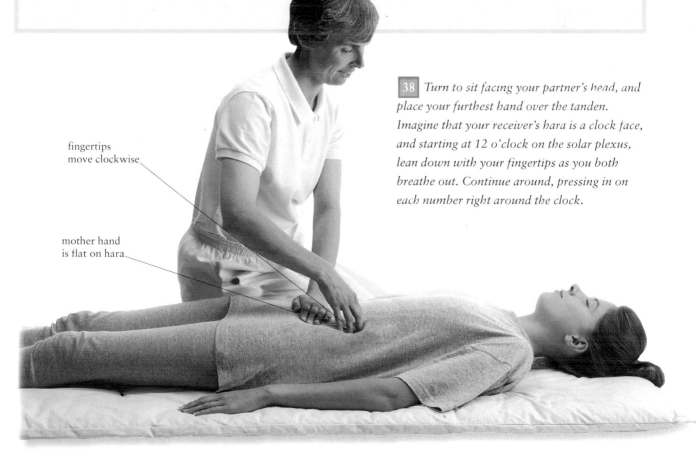

fingertips move clockwise

mother hand is flat on hara

38 *Turn to sit facing your partner's head, and place your furthest hand over the tanden. Imagine that your receiver's hara is a clock face, and starting at 12 o'clock on the solar plexus, lean down with your fingertips as you both breathe out. Continue around, pressing in on each number right around the clock.*

The Chest

Working the chest generally can be very useful for relaxation, putting your receiver in touch with his or her breathing and allowing the person to focus on his or her more personal and emotional Yin side. Traditionally, the Spleen, Stomach, Liver, and Kidney meridians all pass through the chest, while Heart and Heart Governor begin in the armpit and beside the nipple respectively, with Lung starting below the outer end of the collarbone. In Zen Shiatsu theory, extensions of the Heart and Heart Governor meridians run on the sternum and above the breasts, all of which makes the chest a rich area for dealing with heart and lung conditions, breathing difficulties, and emotional problems.

WORKING THE CHEST

Many people feel vulnerable having the chest worked; however, when you are more experienced you will find that an emotional reaction on the part of your partner can leave the person feeling lighter and more balanced. When working anywhere on the chest, be aware of directing your pressure between the ribs, and be sensitive, because ribs are often tender. Avoid anything but the lightest pressure on breast tissue. The technique used when working the chest will depend to a a large extent on the physical structure of the receiver. General stimulation can be given to everyone using the sides of the hands, as in step 39. If your partner is fairly flat in the chest, you could alternatively use gentle pressure with your palm or the flat of your fingers. More specific meridian stimulation with the thumbs, described in step 40, could also be done with fingertips, one side at a time, with mother hand either on the solar plexus or heart chakras.

> **CAUTION**
> Use light pressure with focused Ki when working on people who have heart or chest problems, or respiratory disorders. Be aware that this is a very personal area and some receivers may find pressure challenging.

MERIDIAN

The Conception Vessel in the center of the chest, and the Kidney meridian just to the outside of the sternum, are the focus of basic work on the ribcage. In addition, once you are more experienced, the supplementary Heart and Heart Governor meridians from Zen Shiatsu can be used to great effect in emotional conditions. Supplementary meridians were identified by Shizuto Masunaga (see p. 28) and provide the practitioner with greater scope to manipulate Ki within the whole body. Supplementary Heart Governor runs along the same course as Conception Vessel, from the solar plexus to CV17 (in line with the nipples), and then branches across the upper breasts to its traditional starting point, one thumb's width out from the nipple. Supplementary Heart runs on the sternum close to HG and then branches above the breast tissue to the armpit.

CAUTION

Work on specific meridians in this area may elicit an emotional release such as weeping or anger from your partner.

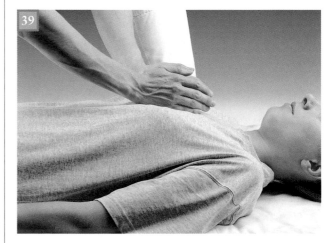

Using the side of your hands, work up the sternum three times. First, work the midline to stimulate the Conception Vessel and supplementary HG. Second, work on the edge of the sternum to cover supplementary HT. Third, stimulate just off the sternum on traditional KD.

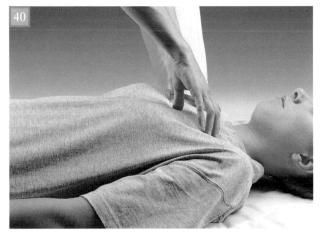

Place your thumbs in the spaces between the ribs at the base of the ribcage. Proceed up the ribcage, holding into each space close to the sternum. Once you reach the collarbone, continue outwards until you reach the hollow before the shoulder joint. One thumb's width down is LU1. Advanced technique: Following the locations described above, work with your thumbs up and out the Heart and Heart Governor supplementary meridians.

41 *Place your nearside hand on your partner's shoulder and hold the wrist with your other hand. Now, supporting the shoulder joint, firmly raise the receiver's arm above the head and stretch upward.*

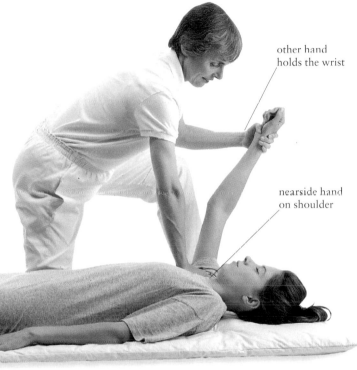

other hand
holds the wrist

nearside hand
on shoulder

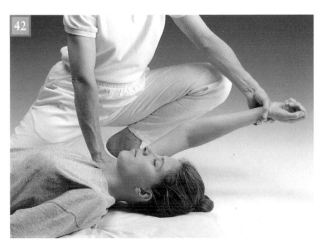

Keeping your support hand on the shoulder, bring the arm out to the side and turn it over so that the back of the hand is uppermost.

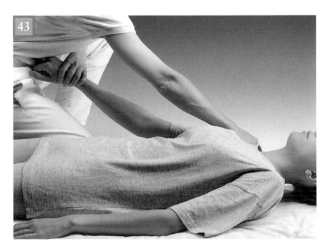

Stretch the arm downward, keeping your grip the same with both of your hands. Go back to step 41 and repeat several times. Once you get the hang of it, this makes a lovely fluid rotation and stretch, which loosens up the shoulder and chest muscles.

Arm Yin Meridians

The Yin meridians of the arm are located on its soft inner surface and are most easily accessed with the arm stretched out with the palm uppermost. In less mobile receivers where the elbow is stiff, you may want to pad under the forearm with a pillow to encourage relaxation. As with the legs, stretch positions are used to make the meridian location clearer: with the arm in treatment position the meridian runs on the most exposed surface. Thus the position for Heart Governor is with the arm straight out horizontally, the Lung position is down at four o'clock or eight o'clock, and the Heart stretch is with the arm bend and hand above the head. This last position may be difficult for some people if they are stiff in the shoulders; in which case you may have to slip your knee under their elbow to support it.

WORKING ARM YIN MERIDIANS

The arm meridians are much closer together than the leg ones, and if you find their location hard to start with, you can just lay the arm into HG (Heart Governor) stretch position and palm the whole inner surface from the shoulder to the fingers, which will cover all three Yin meridians at once. When working the arms, place your mother hand on the shoulder, or if appropriate, on the chest at the level of CV17.

MERIDIAN

The Heart meridian runs from the center of the armpit along a line between the biceps and triceps to the crease on the inner side of the elbow, continuing on the soft skin heading over the wrist and toward the inside of the little finger. In addition to affecting the heart and circulation, working the HT is particularly good for calming the mind and easing emotional ups and downs. There are several useful tsubo, too. HT1, in the center of the armpit, helps pain in the arm, while HT9, at the other extreme on the tip of the little finger, relieves extreme anxiety and can also be used to restore consciousness. The Heart Governor meridian begins just to the outside of the nipple, running down the middle of the arm to the middle finger. Again, several points here are good for anxiety and circulatory problems, while HG6 (two fingers' width above the wrist crease and between the tendons) is especially useful for nausea and vomiting.

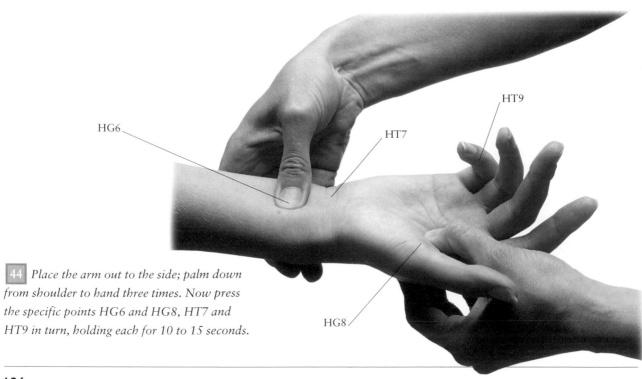

HG6

HT7

HT9

HG8

44 *Place the arm out to the side; palm down from shoulder to hand three times. Now press the specific points HG6 and HG8, HT7 and HT9 in turn, holding each for 10 to 15 seconds.*

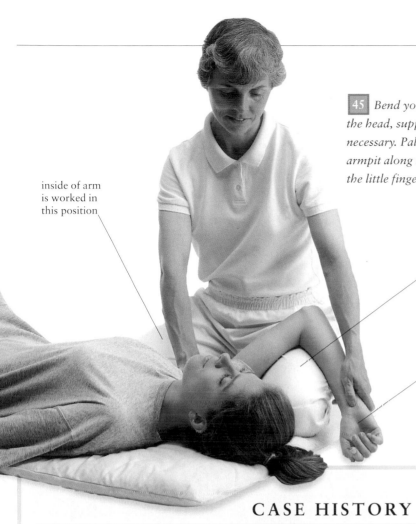

inside of arm
is worked in
this position

arm is supported by
practitioner's thigh

hand is
above head

45 *Bend your partner's arm so that the hand is above the head, supporting the elbow with your knee, if necessary. Palm, then thumb, HT from the inside of the armpit along the bottom edge of the arm to the inside of the little finger.*

CASE HISTORY

Mrs. L., female, 55 years

Mrs. L. initially came for treatment for menopausal symptoms, which included hot flushes, night sweats, and heavy legs with fluid retention. Generally her emotional and mental state was quite stable when she came for her session, although she did complain of mood swings. Despite intermittent problems with self-esteem, she is always beautifully made up with hair carefully arranged.

PRESENTING SYMPTOMS: On this particular occasion, Mrs. L. was very upset and feeling unfairly treated by the college where she was doing a course. She had not been allowed to take the end-of-year exam because she had not completed the homework assignments, which was partly to do with work and family stress, and partly to do with difficulties she experienced in studying.

DIAGNOSIS: SP kyo, HT jitsu.

ANALYSIS: This was a departure from the usual KD kyo pattern related to her menopausal problems. It was obvious to me that today the diagnosis had to be interpreted in emotional and psychological terms, since she was so upset. Psychologically, the Spleen meridian is to do with thoughts, intellectual activity, and sense of self; since she had been studying hard and doing a great deal of thinking about her place and role in society, she had depleted Spleen function, to the extent that the emotional aspect, sympathy, had turned in upon herself into a "poor me" attitude. Heart jitsu often appears when there is excessive emotional activity, often with a sense of overreacting. Although she seemed to be calmer after talking about the problem, there was still an underlying feeling of mental agitation that fitted in with HT jitsu.

TREATMENT: I spent the first part of the session working on the chest to calm the emotional centers. Supplementary HT meridian was used in conjunction with her breathing pattern (step 40, advanced technique), as well as CV17, which has the effect of resolving tightness in the chest and calming the emotions. This was followed by work on the traditional Heart meridian in the arms, paying particular attention to points HT7 and HT9 in order to calm the mind (steps 44 and 45). I then worked on the Spleen meridian in the legs to balance the deficiency and to take Ki down and away from the chest. She felt much more at peace after the session.

Arm Yin Meridians and Hand Massage

When palming along the Yin meridians, be careful to avoid strong pressure on the elbow joint, since this can be uncomfortable. Make sure you have sufficient padding under the wrist and hands to ensure the receiver's comfort – if you are just using a blanket rather than a futon or mat, palm more gently on the hands or place cushions under the arms and hands while you work them.

WORKING THE HANDS

The hands, like the feet, are used and abused so often, yet they are rarely given much attention. Begin the hand sequence as if shaking hands while supporting the wrist with your other hand. Rotate three times in each direction, then stretch forward and backward. Now spread the palm open with sweeping thumb movements. Work with your thumb on the palm, in between the bones, and then turn the hand over and work the back in the same way, between the bones from wrist to fingers. Holding each finger in turn firmly near its base, rotate them singly in both directions and then squeeze down the sides to the nail bed. This stimulates the beginnings and endings of the meridians that run through the arms.

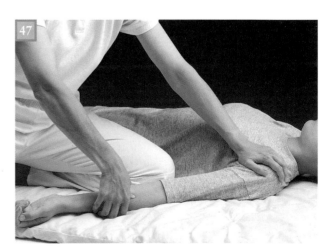

MERIDIAN

The Lung meridian completes the Yin trio in the arm. Its first point is to be found one thumb's width down from the hollow under the outer end of the collar bone; LU2 is in that hollow. The meridian then flows along the upper side of the biceps through the elbow, toward the thumb side of the hand. The Lung meridian obviously governs breathing on a physical level: psychologically and emotionally, it has to do with structure and boundaries, positivity, and melancholy, or depression. Lung tsubo are almost all involved in some way in the treatment of respiratory conditions such as asthma or bronchitis. Our intake of Air Ki is governed by the Lung meridian, therefore in cases of tiredness and not taking in enough new Ki, it is useful to work the Lung meridian and asking your receiver to breathe consciously in rhythm with your pressure.

Place the arm straight out to the side. Palm and then thumb right along the middle for the Heart Governor, remembering to hold HG6 and 8 for 10 to 15 seconds.

Angle the arm farther down (at four o'clock or eight o'clock) for the Lung meridian, and palm then thumb along the upper surface of the biceps, ending on the palm side of the thumb.

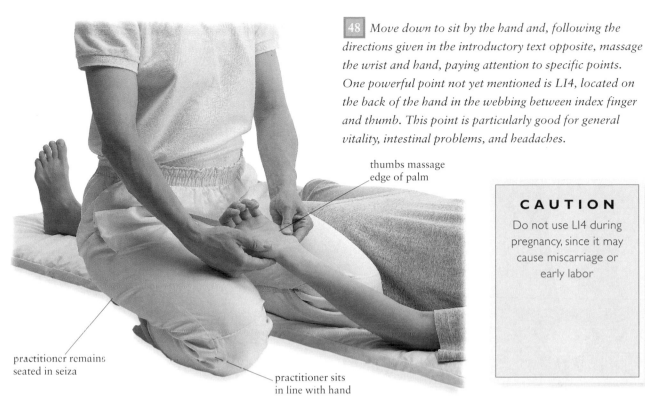

48 *Move down to sit by the hand and, following the directions given in the introductory text opposite, massage the wrist and hand, paying attention to specific points. One powerful point not yet mentioned is LI4, located on the back of the hand in the webbing between index finger and thumb. This point is particularly good for general vitality, intestinal problems, and headaches.*

thumbs massage
edge of palm

practitioner remains
seated in seiza

practitioner sits
in line with hand

CAUTION

Do not use LI4 during pregnancy, since it may cause miscarriage or early labor

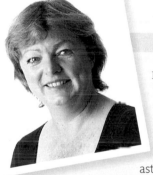

CASE HISTORY
Mrs. B., female, 45 years

PRESENTING SYMPTOMS: Mrs. B. came for treatment whenever her asthma was particularly bad. Because of the large amount of medication she was on for this condition, she also tended to suffer from depression. One of the drugs she took in inhaler form caused headaches, and she was generally very stiff in the neck and shoulders.

MEDICAL HISTORY: Severe allergic asthma since early childhood; sensitive to many substances, resulting in coughing and wheezing. The latter symptoms were also worse on exertion, on change of temperature, and in humid conditions.

ANALYSIS: Dry skin and congested nose combined with the other symptoms to form a pattern in which the Metal Element is compromised and the Lung meridian is unable to fulfill its traditional function of protecting the body's Ki from external factors such as Heat, Dryness, Wind, and so on.

DIAGNOSIS: There was a pattern of LU or LI kyo combined with LV or GB jitsu.

TREATMENT: Because her symptoms involved both the physical aspect (asthma) and the psychological aspect (depression) of Lung, and its wider function of allowing the intake and elimination of Ki, I found that concerted work on the Lung meridian (step 47) was useful. In addition, I usually worked extensively on the hands, since this has a relaxing effect and she particularly enjoyed the feel of LI4 being stimulated (step 48). LI4 is a powerful point in relieving headaches, which were also part of her symptom pattern. The Gall Bladder meridian is related to muscular stiffness, especially in the neck muscles, and we regularly worked tender points on the meridian to disperse tightness, often with very good effect.

Arm Yang Meridians

The arm Yang meridians originate in the fingers and flow downward along the arms to the shoulders, and up the neck to finish on the head. If you remember that Yang energy flows from Heaven down, and Yin energy from Earth upward, it will help you to recall that the numbering of the Yang meridians goes from fingers to head. However, in the Zen Shiatsu method, the Ki flow can be balanced by working from the hara outward, so the arm Yang channels are stimulated from shoulder to fingertips.

WORKING ARM YANG MERIDIANS

As with other meridians, stretch positions make location easier. The treatment position for Large Intestine is similar to its pair, Lung, but with the Yang back surface uppermost. Triple Heater is worked with the arm across the waist. Small Intestine is the third arm Yang meridian; place the arm across the chest with the hand on the opposite shoulder. From here you can thumb effectively all the way to the little finger.

CAUTION

Do not press LI4 during pregnancy, since it may cause early labor or miscarriage.

MERIDIAN

Small Intestine is a little complex in the head, neck, and shoulder, but thereafter runs a simple course down the back of the arm from the armpit crease to the inner elbow crease, then along the outside back of the arm to the outside of the little finger. Its function is assimilation on all levels, physically with regard to food, and mentally with regard to information, experiences, and emotions. The Triple Heater function has already been covered in some depth. It runs from the rear dimple that appears when the deltoid muscle is abducted, down the middle of the upper arm, over the elbow, and then between the radius and ulna bones to the outside of the fourth finger. Large Intestine can be found in the front dimple at the top of the deltoid, running to the outer end of the elbow crease, along the prominent muscle to the front of the forearm, into LI4 in the webbing between index finger and thumb, and then to the index finger itself.

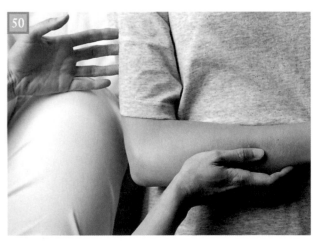

Pick up the arm and give it a little shake to relax it. Place across the chest, then thumb the upper portion from the end of the armpit crease to the inner elbow crease, then along the back of the ulna bone to the little finger.

Place the arm across the waist. Use your outstretched fingertips to stimulate from the rear portion of deltoid to the point of the elbow, then between the radius and ulna along to the fourth finger.

CASE HISTORY
Mr. J., male, 45 years

PRESENTING SYMPTOMS: Mr. J. came with severe pain in his left shoulder, which he had been experiencing for several months. He described the pain as like a toothache, a bony pain rather than a muscular one, and more or less constant, although worse after heavy lifting. An X-ray had revealed thinning of the bone and some arthritic changes in the shoulder joint where the deltoid muscle originates.

MEDICAL HISTORY: There was nothing in Mr. J.'s case history that produced pointers to any particular meridian or Element imbalance. He was generally in good health with a sensible diet and positive outlook.

BACKGROUND: Part of Mr. J.'s work involved carrying a heavy item, which he invariably did with the left arm bent and held away from his body. In other words, he used the deltoid muscle, which is located at the top of the arm and whose function is to raise the arm away from the body.

DIAGNOSIS AND ANALYSIS: Kidney meridian showed up kyo in his first three treatments; however, I felt that the left shoulder pain was more in the nature of a localized problem in this case, directly attributable to repetitive strain injury rather than meridian imbalance.

The pain he was experiencing was due to chronic tension in the fibers of the deltoid muscle, which had become incapable of relaxing again after being overused in the course of his work.

TREATMENT: In general, his shoulders were very tight, so I concentrated initially on loosening by working the trapezius muscle (steps 7 to 9) on both sides. I also worked on the supplementary KD meridian in the arms and traditional KD in the leg, to balance his Ki and draw energy away from the shoulders by working the feet. The main part of the treatments were spent working directly on the site of pain, particularly on the excessive muscle tone in the front portion of deltoid. Working the Large Intestine meridian in the shoulder and arm was useful (step 51), as was friction rubbing across the muscle fibers and pressing tsubo LI15 and TH14 (in the hollows formed at the top of deltoid when the muscle is activated). Since I also wanted to increase local circulation, I applied indirect moxa to these points to heat up the area, energize blocked Ki, and mobilize the shoulder joint. After four sessions the condition had gone except for the occasional twinge.

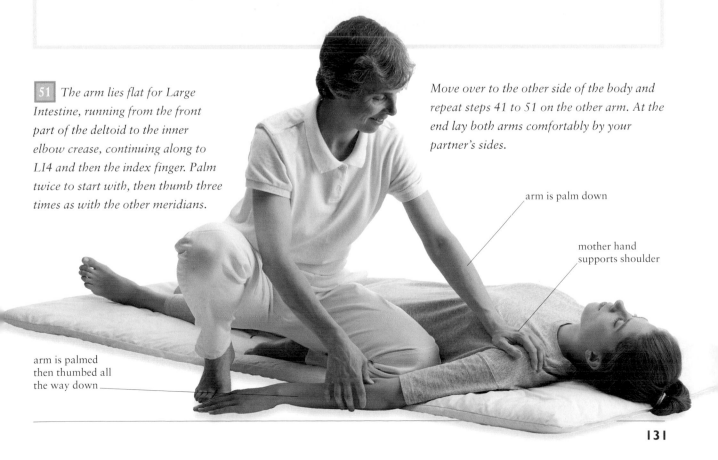

51 *The arm lies flat for Large Intestine, running from the front part of the deltoid to the inner elbow crease, continuing along to LI4 and then the index finger. Palm twice to start with, then thumb three times as with the other meridians.*

Move over to the other side of the body and repeat steps 41 to 51 on the other arm. At the end lay both arms comfortably by your partner's sides.

arm is palm down

mother hand supports shoulder

arm is palmed then thumbed all the way down

Neck and Head

Many people have a tendency to hold much of their energy in the head and neck; it's well-known that tension manifests itself in this area. Neck muscles in particular can become very tight and block the flow of Ki to and from the rest of the body, resulting in headaches, migraines, or dizzy sensations. In the front of the neck the sternocleidomastoid muscle (SCM), which is the prime mover in turning the head from side to side, is crossed by the Stomach, Large Intestine, and Small Intestine meridians.

WORKING THE NECK AND HEAD

Although you should always be careful working the front of the neck, since there are important arteries, veins, and nerves located there, gentle squeezing down the fibers of the SCM, as in step 57 (opposite), can be extremely effective in preventing and reducing head and neck pain.

Lengthening the neck by gentle traction from the base of the skull helps the whole of the spine to relax and stretch out, while safe and effective side stretches on the neck are made by holding the head at an angle and pushing the shoulder away.

MERIDIAN

The neck and head contain several important meridians, and their pathways are complex and intertwining. The Bladder meridian begins at the inside corner of the eyes and flows over the top of the head to run close to the spine down the neck and back. The Bladder meridian actually finishes on the little toe and has no less than 67 tsubo, but BL1 and BL2 (the inner corner of the eye and on the upper eye socket respectively) help with eye problems and headaches. Gall Bladder has a complex zigzag pathway beginning at the outer corner of the eye and sweeping over the head three times before descending the neck. Triple Heater has its final point at the outside end of the eyebrow, passes close around the ear, and then runs down toward the back of the shoulder. In addition, the Governing Vessel runs centrally from the spine to the crown and the forehead before going deep into the body through the mouth.

52 *Kneeling above your partner's head, place your fingertips at the base of the skull and draw the head toward you by leaning back. This puts gentle traction on the whole spine.*

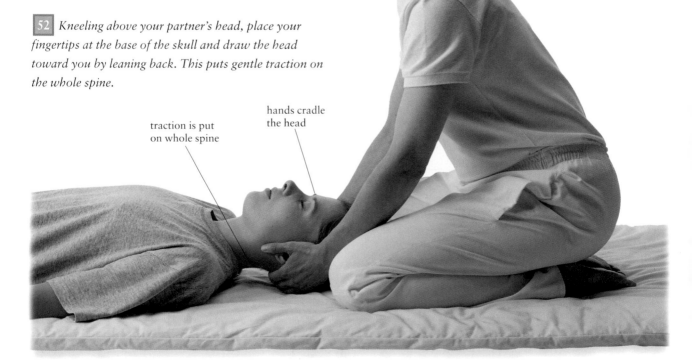

traction is put
on whole spine

hands cradle
the head

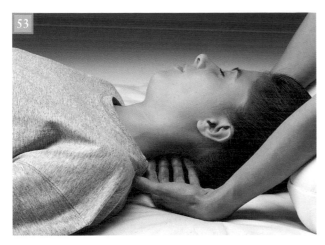

Beginning just outside the large muscles at the back of the neck, press upward with middle fingers, working close to the spine. Stimulate from the skull to the top of the back.

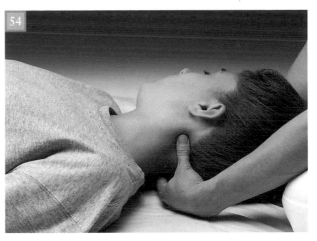

Turn the head to one side and stimulate GB20, which is found in the hollow between the two large neck muscles – trapezius and sternocleidomastoid.

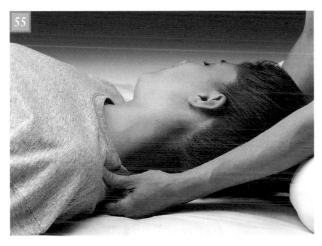

From GB20, thumb down the side of the neck along the top of the shoulder muscle until you meet the shoulder joint. Caution: If your partner is pregnant, avoid GB21 on top of the shoulder.

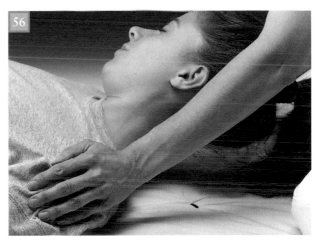

Advanced technique: Cradle the head with the face turned to the side. As your partner breathes out, create a stretch by pushing the shoulder down toward the feet.

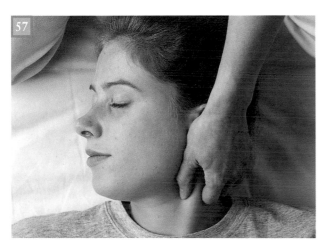

Advanced technique: Gently squeeze both sides of the SCM muscle from just behind the ear to the inner end of the collarbone. Turn the head and repeat steps 54 to 57.

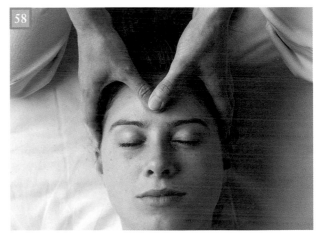

Center your receiver's head. Putting one thumb on top of the other, work from between the eyebrows up the center of the forehead to the top of the crown.

3 Completing the Basic Sequence

Traditionally, all six Yang meridians either begin or end in the head. Although the traditional flows are both up and down the neck, in practice it is found to be more effective to work down from the head, as this encourages energy "stuck" in the head and neck to disperse into the rest of the body.

This facial routine is a simple sequence following the bone structures of the face and stimulating points for relieving head pain, toothaches, and sinus problems, and generally promoting relaxation. Shiatsu treatments usually finish on the face, whether the practitioner is a beginner or an experienced practitioner. This is because it is very nurturing and relaxing to have the face worked gently. Always keep your pressure light and your fingers relaxed; this encourages your partner to let go and drift off.

At the end of the session, at the "Third Eye" between the eyebrows and the tanden in the center of the hara, move away quietly, cover your receiver gently with a blanket if appropriate, and go and wash your hands.

MERIDIAN

Stomach, Large, and Small Intestine meridians are located principally in the face and front of the neck, although Small Intestine swings over into this area from the back of the shoulders. Level with the tip of the larynx (Adam's apple) on either side of the SCM muscle, there are two points (ST9 the inner and LI18 the outer), which can be squeezed and stimulated at the same time, and these are very useful for sore throats and neck pain respectively (see step 57). ST3 under the cheekbone can be good for facial paralysis and neuralgia, while pressing the end point of Large Intestine, LI20, helps with sinus pain and stuffy noses. Small Intestine also has points on the cheek which may be used for neuralgia or hearing problems.

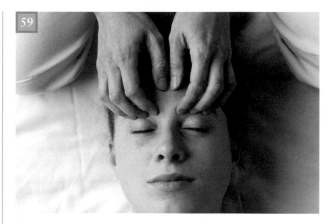

Work around the line of the eye socket, using the fingertips at the top and the thumbs on the lower border. Be careful not to drag the skin.

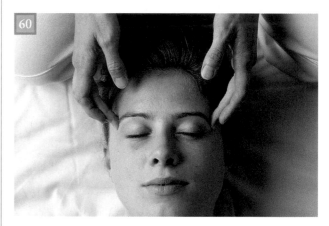

Stimulate down the sides of the nose and out along the cheekbones. Gently press around the lips, over the teeth, then squeeze along the lower jaw with thumb and index finger. Work on specific points such as ST3 as appropriate.

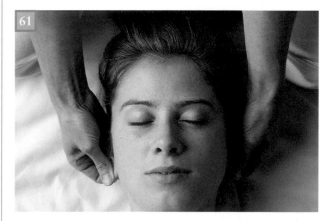

Using your index finger and thumb, massage all over the ears, and pull the earlobes down toward the shoulders.

62 *Move back to sit by your partner's hara. To balance the major energy centers, use the lightest touch and place a thumb at the "Third Eye" just between the eyebrows, and the other at the tanden, three fingers' width below the navel. Hold for 10 seconds as you take three deep, slow breaths into your hara, then allow your thumbs to float off the body.*

63 *Sit quietly based in hara for a moment or two as you mentally "finish off" the session. Cover your partner with a blanket if that seems necessary, then go and wash your hands in order to completely break contact, physically and mentally, with your partner's Ki. You should also make a point of taking three or four deep breaths to recharge your own Ki.*

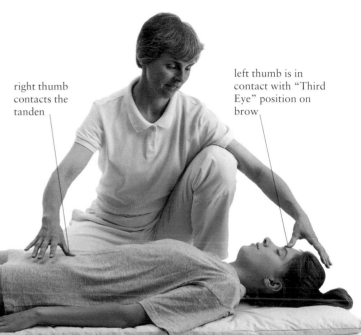

right thumb contacts the tanden

left thumb is in contact with "Third Eye" position on brow

CASE HISTORY
Mrs. C., female, 40 years

PRESENTING SYMPTOMS: Mrs. C. arrived for her first treatment with severe neck pain on the right-hand side. She had been in a car accident five days earlier and had suffered whiplash, although the bad pain had not commenced until three days later. Prior to the accident she had spent the day stripping wallpaper in an awkward position over a bathtub and had felt some tension in her neck.

MEDICAL HISTORY: On HRT following hysterectomy, indigestion, sleep disturbance due to road works outside her house, general stiffness in neck and shoulders. Stress in home and family life.

DIAGNOSIS: LI kyo, HT jitsu for the first two treatments, changing to ST kyo, GB jitsu, then long-term pattern KD kyo, LI jitsu.

TREATMENT: As the neck was so sore, I decided to focus upon it first in the session, and used very gentle traction (step 52) to start the relaxation process. Since this was the kyo meridian, working BL and GB in the neck (steps 53 and 55), as well as LI, eased the pain somewhat. I followed this with some very focused work on the SCM muscle (step 57), since this is commonly affected in whiplash. Having prepared the neck in this way I was then able to do some side stretches (step 56) very gently at several different angles to ease out different neck muscles. Heart meridian was then worked in the arm, since I felt there was some emotional trauma involving the accident that needed to be resolved; HT points also help with sleep disturbance.

After the first two treatments using this pattern, she reported feeling a lot better with no pain and having more movement than for a long time. In the next session we worked quite a bit on the jitsu GB and ST meridian in the neck. By the fourth treatment we were past the initial neck problem and starting to work with more long-term imbalances.

4 Simple One-Handed Hara Diagnosis

Once you have become accustomed to giving the basic Shiatsu sequence laid out in this section, you may want to start homing in on particular meridians to help rebalance certain health conditions. By using the table of meridian associations and imbalances on pages 70–73, and the simplified form of hara diagnosis that follows, we can make a reasonably accurate diagnosis using the kyo-jitsu model, which can then be applied to your basic sequence by simply concentrating more on the specified meridians and leaving out other parts of the form. I would stress that this is not a full Shiatsu diagnosis and if you want to learn properly you should arrange to go to Shiatsu classes. You cannot really learn any hands-on practical skill in any depth from a book – much better to have a qualified person by your side to guide you.

Look back to the hara diagnostic areas map on page 75. Sit in seiza beside your partner facing his or her head with your thigh making contact with the side of the body. Using a relaxed hand and fairly light touch, feel each of the areas in turn with the hand nearest your partner to see how far your fingertips sink into his or her hara at each position. The secret here is to keep your fingers very loose and angle them so that you are going straight in at 90 degrees. Imagine you are dipping your fingertips slowly into a bowl of water to see how hot it is. What we are feeling for is kyo or jitsu quality: does the area feel loose or tight, yielding or resistant, soft or bouncy? Rather than pressing in, try to rest your fingers on the surface of the hara and note how far the hara allows you to sink in. If there is no resistance or reaction or if it feels very soft, that is a kyo feeling. Jitsu feels firmer or bouncy and definitely responds to your touch.

Now go through all the areas again in the same way and try to pinpoint which area feels the most kyo and which the most jitsu. The order that we generally use to go through the hara areas is HT, GB, LIV, right LU, ST, TH, left LU, HT, HG, SP (use the flat of your fingers so as not to pick up the pulse), KD, BL, left LI, right LI, left SI, right SI. By going around the areas in the same order (which is, by the way, merely a convention), we get into a routine that allows us to concentrate on what we are feeling, not where we are going next or whether we have missed out any of the areas.

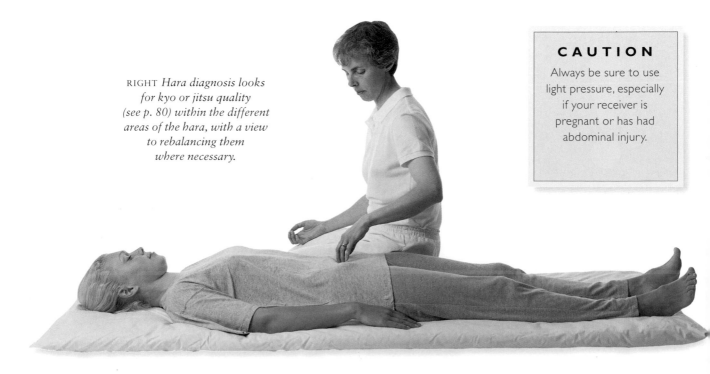

RIGHT *Hara diagnosis looks for kyo or jitsu quality (see p. 80) within the different areas of the hara, with a view to rebalancing them where necessary.*

CAUTION

Always be sure to use light pressure, especially if your receiver is pregnant or has had abdominal injury.

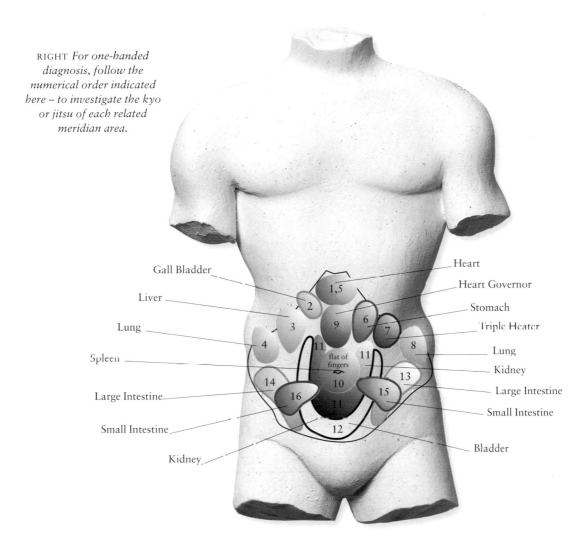

RIGHT *For one-handed diagnosis, follow the numerical order indicated here – to investigate the kyo or jitsu of each related meridian area.*

Gall Bladder

Liver

Lung

Spleen

Large Intestine

Small Intestine

Kidney

Heart

Heart Governor

Stomach

Triple Heater

Lung

Kidney

Large Intestine

Small Intestine

Bladder

flat of fingers

The diagnostic areas that feel most kyo and most jitsu correspond to the meridians that are most out of balance, and therefore, once you have found them, you can give them more attention in your session. Usually we spend more time on tonifying the kyo, since this is seen as the cause of imbalance.

If, on palpating the hara, you find several areas feel kyo and, say, one or two definitely jitsu, you can try the more advanced technique of "finding the connection" between kyo and jitsu areas. This determines which is the combination most in need of rebalancing. Bearing in mind that kyo and jitsu are in an energetic relationship, one of the areas you felt as jitsu will react in some way (often by relaxing or softening) as you palpate one of the kyo areas. The method is therefore to hold lightly one jitsu area, and with the other hand dip more deeply into each of your kyo areas in turn. If you feel a reaction in your jitsu hand, then you have found the kyo-jitsu meridian imbalance that is manifesting right now. If you don't feel any reaction, then go to your next jitsu area and repeat the process. Bear in mind that this is an advanced technique requiring greater sensitivity, so you may not find the reacting pair quite as easily as just looking for a "most kyo" or a "most jitsu." Also remember that Ki can change quickly in hara, so the longer you spend dipping into the kyo areas, the more likely you are to start subconsciously treating them so the diagnostic pattern will change.

Over a period of time, if you work on someone regularly, you will start to see patterns emerging in diagnosis, which, if you note them and look up their theoretical associations, will show you how theory and practice correlate and work together in concert. This is the real start of your journey of understanding into the fascinating world of the workings of Ki.

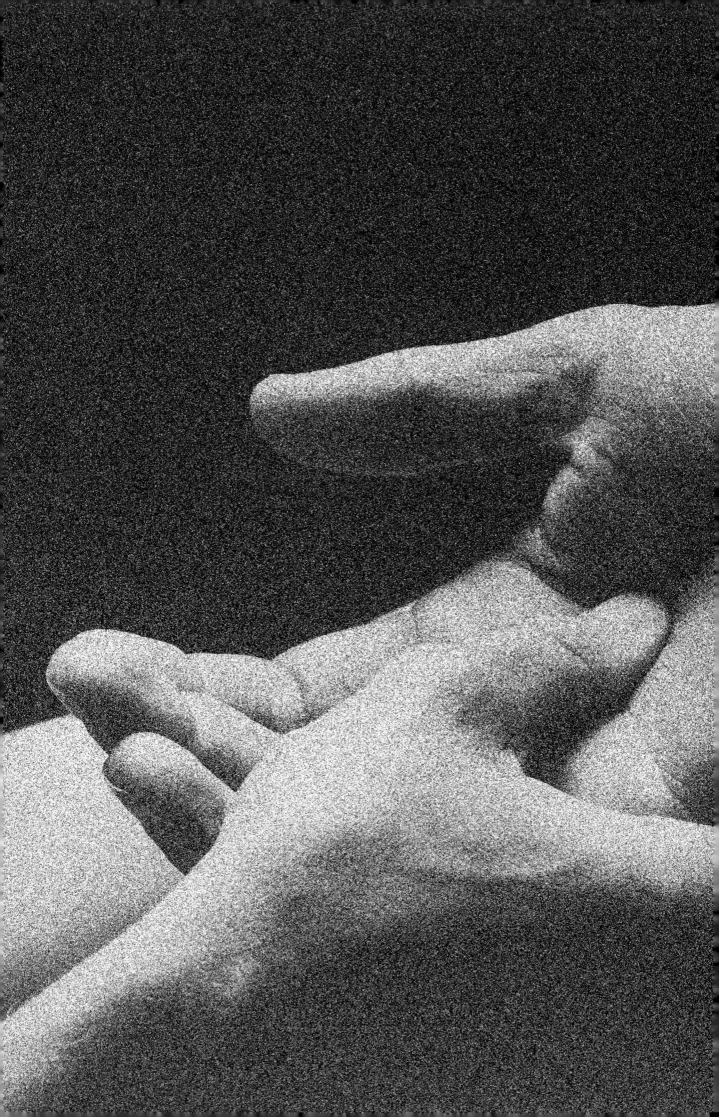

RELATED EXERCISES AND SELF-HELP MEASURES

Students of Shiatsu can improve their ability to help others and their own well-being through the regular practice of some simple exercises.

1 The Shiatsu Lifestyle

For me, and for many practitioners, giving Shiatsu is not just about applying a set of techniques to a body; it is a whole way of living and being. It is a physical and spiritual discipline that allows me to give to others while at the same time developing my Self.

Having a knowledge and direct experience of Ki, I tend to look at what happens to me and to those around me in terms of energy. It is as if the theories of Yin and Yang, Five Elements, and kyo-jitsu have become a personal map that helps me to interpret not just events in my immediate circle, but phenomena in the wider world, too. I find it fascinating to be consciously aware of the interplay of Ki, certainly when I am working on someone's sore shoulder or painful back, but also when I observe my students working on each other, when I have to chair a meeting in which there is some conflict, or when I watch my daughter riding her pony. It is also apparent when you read in the newspaper of some global event or political development. On a much wider scale, what is happening in the Ki of collective consciousness when a country votes one party of government out and another in? What is happening to the Ki of the earth when there are volcanoes erupting and floods causing devastation?

Being aware of Ki can allow us to look upon diverse events with different eyes, and in regard to our own lives can give us an element of control. For example, this morning I was getting very frustrated, dominated by Yang and the element of Wood, not seeing how I was to accomplish all the things I needed to do in a short space of time. A five minute break to stand back, do some deep breathing, and structure my day, in Metallic mode, has enabled me to come back to a measure of balance and get down to work without becoming too frustrated.

RIGHT *Physical exercise helps to balance out the modern lifestyle that is so often dominated by sedentary or intellectual work.*

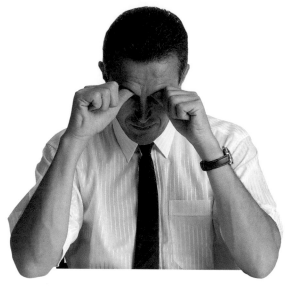

ABOVE *Pressing BL2 in the upper eye socket helps relieve headaches and sore, red eyes.*

THE VALUE OF EXERCISES

Self-help activities and self-development exercises are most effective in creating balance in ourselves and developing the perceptions and sensitivity needed for good Shiatsu. They can connect us consciously with our Ki, open our minds, and stretch our bodies. And they can be fun! One of my favorite "exercises" I give to patients or students – especially those who spend excessive amounts of time doing things for others – is to tell them to have a treat, a challenge, and an adventure every day for a week. Try it yourself, and notice which one of those three you find most difficult.

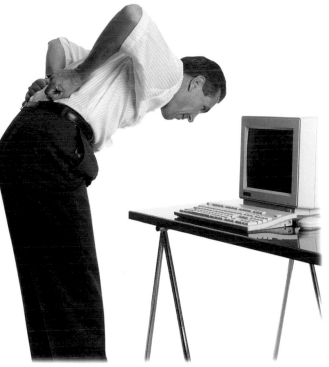

ABOVE *Take a break from the computer and prevent backache by tapping down the Bladder meridian in the back.*

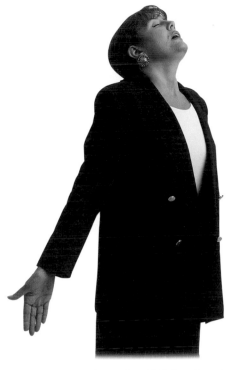

ABOVE *A couple of full deep breaths by an open window can renew your energy after a difficult business meeting.*

The important thing about exercises is that they have to be within the grasp of the person doing them. It is no good expecting the overweight businessman who is constantly pushed for time to go jogging for an hour every lunchtime, or a night bird to get up and do an hour's yoga before breakfast.

Personally, I especially like exercises and self-help measures that can either be done relatively quickly or be incorporated into the day's business. In the past, there were periods when I spent considerable time on my personal development practices: aikido, yoga, meditation, cooking perfectly balanced Yin Yang meals, and other pursuits. Several years ago I was practicing Shiatsu for six or more hours per day as well as teaching Shiatsu nearly every weekend. These days my practice is less busy and my teaching commitments slightly less pressured, my activities are more home-centered, and I find that by being mindful of the principles and workings of Ki, the Shiatsu practice and teaching I do are sufficient spiritual and physical discipline. However, I have many years' experience behind me.

If you are just starting out on the road of Shiatsu and self-understanding, try to take at least half an hour every day on some of these exercises. Spending time alone, just being with ourselves, is important for us all to remind us of who we are especially for those with heavy demands made on them.

The following exercises are simple, can take as much or as little time as you have available, and can really make a difference to the quality of your life.

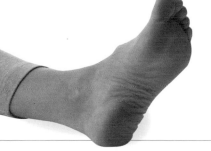

Hara Development and Breathing Exercises

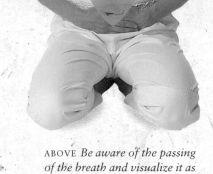

One of the most powerful things we can learn in life is how to be in touch with our hara. In the East it is said that mind and body come together in the hara: here is the center of our physical energy and our mental forces – the very essence of our Self. The first step to being able to harness the power of hara is awareness.

ABOVE *Be aware of the passing of the breath and visualize it as a stream of light.*

A BALL OF LIGHT

Place your fingertips on the tanden, the center of your hara, three fingers'-width below the navel, and press in. Imagine a ball of light there deep inside your body. On and off during the day, remember about this ball of light and just be aware of it as you go about your normal activities. Then next time you have to climb a lot of stairs or run for any length of time, instead of thinking about your tired legs or sore chest, think of the ball of light in your hara; you will find it easier to get to where you want to be.

Using hara is also effective in emotional situations. If you feel yourself becoming angry or frightened take several deep breaths, allowing the breath to expand right down to your hara, and be conscious of your tanden – if necessary, you can even touch it to center yourself. Your anger or fear will now be more controlled and you will feel more distanced from the situation and able to react appropriately.

RIGHT *With the fingertips lightly pressing on the tanden, imagine a ball of light concentrated there.*

A STREAM OF LIGHT

This is one to do quietly for 10 minutes by yourself. Sit comfortably with your spine straight, either on a chair, on the floor cross-legged, or in seiza. Become aware of your hara. As you breathe in through your nose, imagine your breath as a stream of light filling up your hara. Keep the image of light at the hara and let the excess breath slip out through your mouth, so that you create a reservoir of light in your hara that grows stronger with every in-breath. This can be done as an exercise on its own or as a preparation for giving Shiatsu. If you are about to give Shiatsu, you can then extend the exercise by breathing out the stream of light through your hands and into your partner. The light is of course a visualization of Ki.

FILLING THE BODY WITH LIGHT

Again, take a few quiet minutes to yourself. Breathe to center yourself in hara as in the last exercise. Now take a deeper breath and imagine the inflowing Ki filling not just your hara, but the whole of your body. Visualize Ki as light (any color that comes to you naturally or bright white light) and see it expanding from the center of your hara, radiating out to your shoulders, arms, and fingers, to your thighs, knees, and feet. Then, as you exhale, blow the Ki out through your mouth, emptying all the light out until only a little ball remains at your tanden.

These exercises should never cause you any discomfort, so don't hold your breath before exhaling. Simply breathe in deeply, perhaps for a count of eight, to give yourself a chance to visualize the light radiating into your body, then exhale more quickly, for a count of four.

If initially you find it hard to visualize expanding Ki into your whole body, then alternate between filling and emptying the upper body and the lower body.

This is a good exercise if you have been feeling drained or negative, because it allows you to visualize emptying out all the old stale Ki and bringing in new, positive energy to replace it.

A variation of this exercise is to breathe light to any part of your body that is feeling tired, stressed, or painful. Allow the healing light to bathe the area of discomfort and then, on a strong out-breath, visualize the imbalanced Ki being blown away out of your body.

BREATHING A SQUARE

This exercise concentrates more on breathing. It has a calming effect. I call it "breathing a square," because you breathe in to the count of four (as fast or slowly as is comfortable), hold your breath for four, breathe out to the count of four, and again hold for four. As you do this, be aware of your hara and be careful not to let your shoulders come up as you hold the breath. Let the Ki settle down in hara as you hold your breath. At first, don't breathe in, out or hold for longer than a count of four in case you feel faint. However, as you become used to this exercise, you may find in time that you have enough control to increase the counts to six, or even eight.

Variations on "breathing a square" can include making the exhalation twice as long as the inhalation; holding the breath for a count of four at the end of the exhalation; holding the breath at the end of both inhalation and exhalation. So long as you remain focused on your tanden, keeping shoulders and chest relaxed, these exercises can help to promote a tranquil outlook by increasing your oxygen intake.

There are lots of other breathing and hara exercises that you may learn if you go to Shiatsu classes; the ones described above are easy ones that you can start with simply and safely on your own.

LEFT *Sitting in seiza is excellent as a restful position for light-visualization.*

2 Do-in or Self-Shiatsu

Do-In or self-Shiatsu is an energizing routine that can be used at any time of day. There are several different versions with lots of variations, but the one I like is an invigorating tapping routine following the meridians.

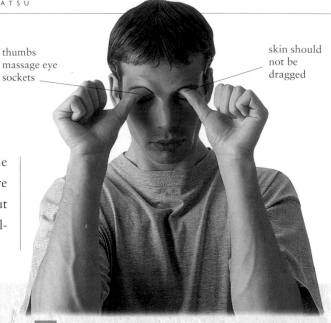

thumbs massage eye sockets

skin should not be dragged

Facial Do-in

Do-in on the head and face area is really good for relieving scalp and facial tension. By tapping the head you can stimulate blood flow to the scalp, promoting healthy hair growth and discharging excess energy. Many of us tense our face muscles unconsciously for much of the time, causing unsightly worry or frown lines on the forehead, while jaw-clenching is a frequent cause of headache. Working around the eyes makes them feel more awake and the pressure activates the lymphatic system, removing toxins that show up so easily in the skin quality of this sensitive area. Nasal congestion and sinus problems can be relieved by pressure at the end of the nostrils and under the cheekbones.

3 *As in the facial Shiatsu routine, stimulate points around your eye socket with your thumbs, being careful not to drag the skin*

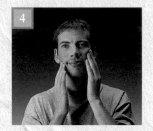

Rub your cheeks and the end of your nose – both actions are good for the circulation.

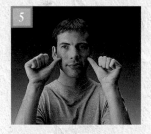

Press into LI20 at the bottom outside corner of the nostrils and then work with thumbs under your cheekbones out as far as your ears.

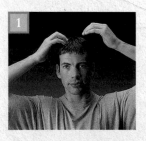

Start by tapping with your fingers on the top of your head. If you keep a loose wrist you can tap quite hard. This exercise helps to wake up the brain in the morning!

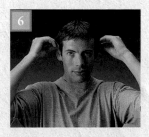

Pull your ears up, down, back and forward, and rub all over – again, good for circulation.

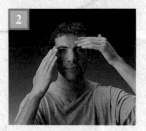

Then smooth across your forehead, followed by making circles at your temples with your fingertips. Squeeze along your eyebrows.

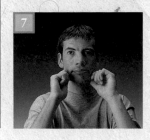

Pinch along the lower jaw, allowing your thumbs to linger on any little nodules or lymph glands so as to squeeze out the toxins.

Neck and Shoulders

All the Yang meridians in the body pass through the neck and shoulders, so stimulating and stretching here is useful to activate them and ensure there is no building of excessive Ki. The neck and shoulders have a complex muscular structure designed to hold up the relatively heavy weight of the head, and are therefore prone to tightness and stress. Stretching and rotating (gently) can release tense muscles as well as promoting Ki flow in the meridians. Be careful, however, if you suffer from spondylitis, osteoporosis, or any other neck problem: for you it is better not to rotate the neck as in Exercise 1, but work a variation of Exercise 2, stretching the neck in each direction and then coming back to center.

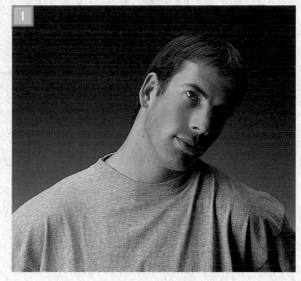

Going as far as you can comfortably, rotate your head in a circle slowly one way and then the other.

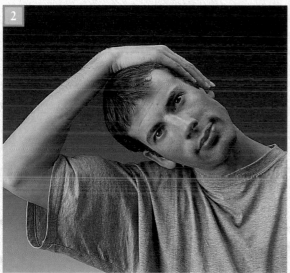

If any position is sore, then place your hand on your head and gently stretch the neck in that place using the weight of your hand to pull the head down.

3 *Making a loose fist, tap on each shoulder in turn. The shoulders often hold a lot of tension, and a good pounding here can release long-held stress.*

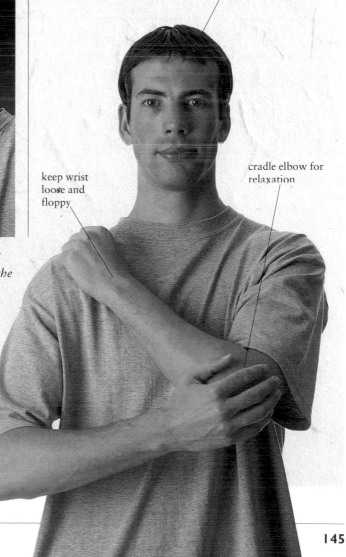

keep head straight

keep wrist loose and floppy

cradle elbow for relaxation

Chest and Arm

Many people tend to collapse the chest forward causing constriction in their breathing and tightness in the pectoral muscles. Tapping here opens the chest and encourages full breathing. Our arms are so often overused; stimulating them dispels tension and prevents the buildup of toxins.

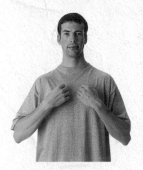

1 *Tap all over your chest (though avoid breast tissue if you are a woman); this can loosen up mucus and make you cough it up. For even greater effect do it with a "Tarzan" yell!*

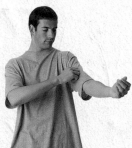

2 *Continue tapping on the arms: up the Yin meridians on the inner arm from shoulder to hand.*

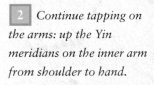

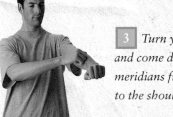

3 *Turn your arm over and come down the Yang meridians from the hand to the shoulder.*

4 *Squeeze and pull each finger in turn and stimulate LI4 and HG8 (look back to the Basic Sequence on page 100 or farther on in this part for the exact locations).*

Back and Leg

The back, buttocks, and thighs are common sites of postural tension that can be alleviated effectively by pounding with a loose wrist.

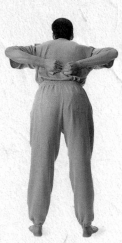

1 *Bend forward and, starting as high up on the back as you can, pummel down either side of the spine from the shoulderblade to buttocks. Again, you can give yourself a good thump if you keep a loose wrist – this stimulates the Bladder meridian.*

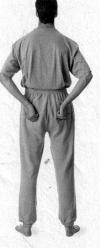

2 *Now pound away on the buttocks to disperse those extra ounces.*

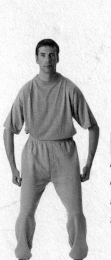

3 *Continuing to tap with a loose fist, work down the outsides of the legs, and up the insides – as always going with the Yin Yang flow.*

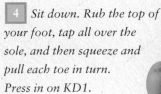

4 *Sit down. Rub the top of your foot, tap all over the sole, and then squeeze and pull each toe in turn. Press in on KD1.*

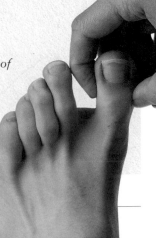

Hara Massage

Getting in touch with your hara is important to help center and ground your energy. Physically mobilizing this area encourages Ki to circulate and ensures that the stagnation so often associated with the abdomen is less likely to occur. You can work on such problems as constipation, indigestion, and menstrual cramps by massaging the hara regularly every day.

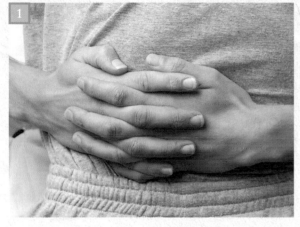

Lie down with your knees bent up. Lacing your fingers together, rock your hara from side to side in the same way as we did in the Shiatsu sequence. Do this for several minutes.

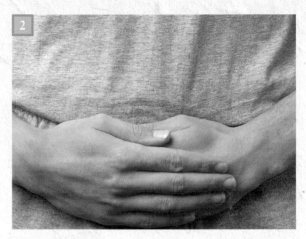

Begin by rocking gently, then go more deeply if this is comfortable. Remember not to rub, but simply to let the intestines move under your hands. Rock lightly before finishing.

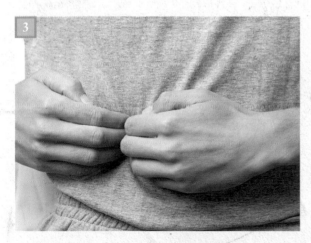

Now starting at the top of the hara at the solar plexus, press inward with your outstretched fingers as you breathe out. Breathe in and move your fingers around to your left, and press in again as you exhale.

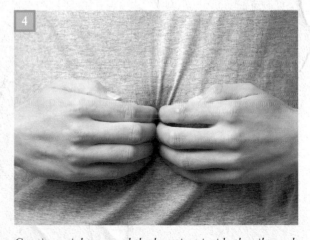

Continue right around the hara just inside the ribs and pelvis for one and a half circuits.

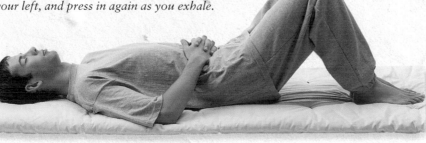

5 *Finally, lay your hands over the tanden and let yourself rest for several minutes.*

3 The Makko-ho Stretches

The Makko-ho stretches are a series of meridian-opening movements that are practiced widely by Shiatsu practitioners and students. They are useful not just because they stretch each pair of meridians, but also because you can monitor the state of your own meridians by the ease and flexibility with which you can get into each position.

Some of the poses are similar to ones used in yoga, but the way of working into them is different. With the Makko-ho exercises, the attitude is a relaxed one: take a breath in, move into the stretch as you breathe out, and relax. Staying in position, breathe in, and as you exhale, try to relax a little further down into the stretch. Don't bounce or try to push yourself into the pose, just go down as far as is comfortable. We usually do three long exhalations for each stretch, and the order in which they are done is in accordance with the Chinese clock cycle (see p. 65).

Each of the Makko-ho exercises stretches a pair of traditional and supplementary (Zen Shiatsu extended) meridians. In addition, the pose either expresses the psychological aspect of the meridian pair or activates a part of the body that is involved in that expression.

Lung/Large Intestine

This stretch opens the chest and focuses on the LU/LI function of "intake of Ki." As well as stretching the LU and LI traditional channels in the arm (especially if the thumbs are linked and index fingers pointed), the supplementary (Zen) LU and LI meridians on the back of the leg are opened by bending forward.

1 *Stand with feet hip-width apart, link your thumbs behind your back.*

link your thumbs behind your back

stand with feet hip-width apart

stretch your arms as far as possible

try to relax down on each exhalation

2 *Bending down, stretch your arms up as far as possible. Breathe in and out three times trying to relax down on each exhalation.*

Stomach/Spleen

The attitude of ST and SP is to do with "grasping food." Imagine someone holding food just out of reach in front of you; or picking up windfall apples; or pulling up carrots – all the emphasis is on the front of the body as you gather the food. The ST/SP stretch takes that front of body concentration of Ki and activates it by stretching the thighs and torso. This is a strenuous exercise so be careful to go only to the stage that is comfortable for you.

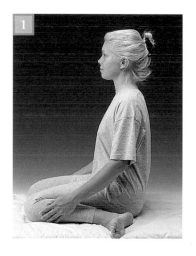

Kneel down with your bottom between your feet. This is similar to sitting in seiza. Feet should be tucked back parallel to the body.

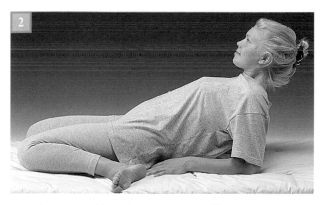

Breathe out, and lean back onto your elbows.

3 *If this is comfortable, on the next exhalation go right down to the floor and raise your hands over your head. Breathe in and out three times.*

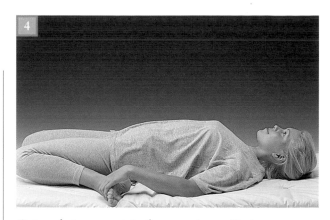

Get ready to come up in the same stages. First, grasp your ankles.

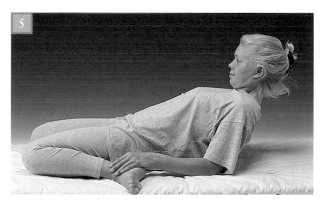

Continuing to grasp your ankles, tucking your chin to chest and push up strongly on your elbows to bring your back off the floor.

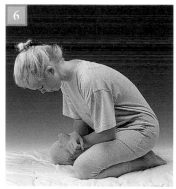

Tuck your feet under your buttocks and then bend forward to counteract the back bend.

7 *If you find this sequence too difficult, sit in seiza, place your hands behind you, breathe out, and raise your hips. Hold for three long breaths to create a stretch on the Stomach and Spleen meridians in the front of the thigh.*

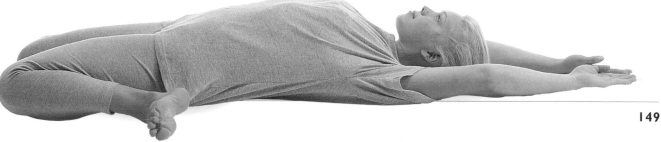

Heart/Small Intestine

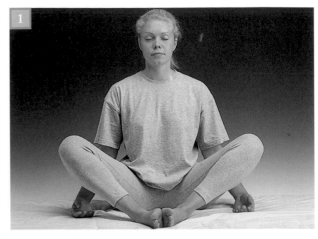

The Heart is the center of awareness, spirituality, and the emotional interpreter of our environment. Small Intestine deals with assimilation, both physically and mentally, in conjunction with the interpretation of the Heart. By sitting in this position, we become more centered and tranquil. Bending forward activates the protected inner surfaces where HT runs, and stretches the Small Intestine pathway.

Sit with the soles of your feet together, drawn up as close to your groin as possible.

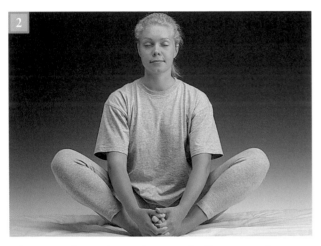

Clasp your feet in front of you, with elbows outside your shins, and relax down toward the floor, trying to keep chest and hara open.

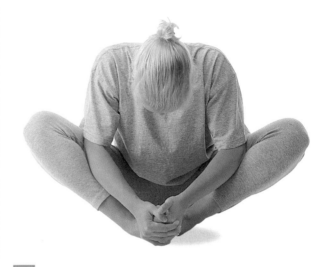

3 *Again, hold the position for three breaths, relaxing down a little on each exhalation.*

Bladder/Kidney

The forward bend of the BL/KD stretch puts you in touch with your back and the back of the legs, aptly expressing the function of "going forward in life" provided by the purification of Bladder and the impetus of Kidney.

1 *With your feet straight out in front of you, bend forward from the hips and push your hands (little fingers uppermost) between your feet if you can reach them. If you can't reach your feet, then hold your ankles or shins just as far as you can go. Breathe and relax down. For the first two breaths look forward between your feet; for the final one, tuck your head down toward your knees to stretch the back of the neck.*

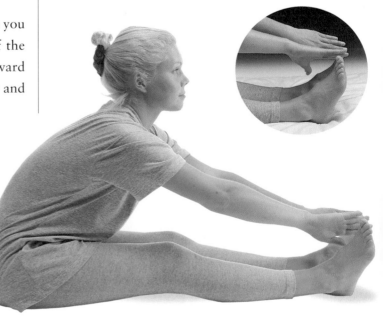

Heart Governor/Triple Heater

This pose embodies the protective attitude of both Heart Governor (also known as Heart Protector) and Triple Heater. It reminds me of a clam shell on the beach, where the harder outer layer, in this case the exposed Triple Heater, protects the soft inner Heart Governor channels.

1 *Sit cross-legged and cross your arms the other way, clasping your knees. Breathe out and stretch forward, pushing your knees down. Again, take three breaths, then reverse legs and arms, and repeat.*

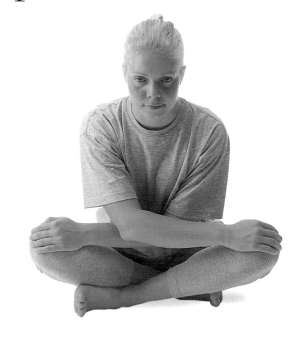

Gall Bladder/Liver

"Which direction to go?" is the physical question being asked in this pose as the sides of the body are stretched first one way and then the other. The Liver's control and planning functions, along with the Gall Bladder's decision-making activities controlling the smooth distribution of Ki, allow us to take action in any given direction. By working this stretch you'll activate these functions in yourself.

1 *Sit with your legs as wide apart as possible, imagining that you have your back to a wall. With your right arm stretched up and your left by your side, stretch down to the left as if sliding down the wall and trying to touch the floor behind your left foot with your right hand. Hold for three breaths.*

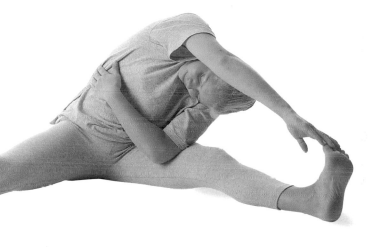

SUMMARY

Although these stretches take no more than five minutes to do, they are a most effective way of keeping you fit and supple, not to mention helping you feel how each pair of meridians is acting in your body. The Makko-ho exercises can be done every morning and night. Remember, however, that you will be stiffer in the morning, and work accordingly.

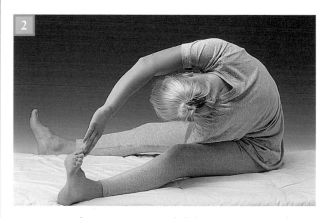

Come up and reverse arms, and slide over to your right in the same way. Remember to keep your back straight and don't collapse your hara. Come back to the center and then, clasping your hands in front of you, bend from the hips straight to the front. Again, take three long breaths as you relax into the stretch.

4 Meditation

Exercises to calm the mind are just as important as physical exercises in Shiatsu. Meditation is the traditional way of stilling the mind and bringing it under control, leading to a sense of peace, well-being, and self-understanding. There are many schools and methods of meditation, all of which have great value. Most of them come from Eastern traditions that are centuries-old and have been brought to the West in recent years. The techniques usually involve breathing exercises, repetition of a sound, visualization, or contemplation of an idea. They are designed to help the mind come to rest so that we can become aware of a deeper, stiller consciousness. When we start on the path of self-development, many of us find that the mind will not be still enough by itself, and therefore I have included four meditation exercises here in which you have to do something.

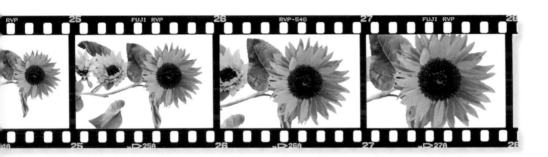

LEFT *A simple meditation exercise is to think about the growth of a plant in terms of freeze-frame photography.*

Natural Meditation

Find an object from nature – a stone, a leaf, or a plant – and place it in front of you. Take five minutes to observe it: pick it up, turn it over, and feel it. Place it down again and imagine where it came from: how a seed grew to form this plant, or how the pebble was ground down from a great rock. Look at all the small details on it. Think about the millions of tiny cells that have divided and developed over time to give that particular leaf its individual shape, color, and texture. If thoughts about other things come into your mind, just let them float away again as you bring your attention back to your object. Do this exercise every day for a week with the same object, then choose a different one.

It is amazing how adults often forget the wonder of the small things in nature. This exercise can bring back that sense of wonder while simultaneously focusing the mind.

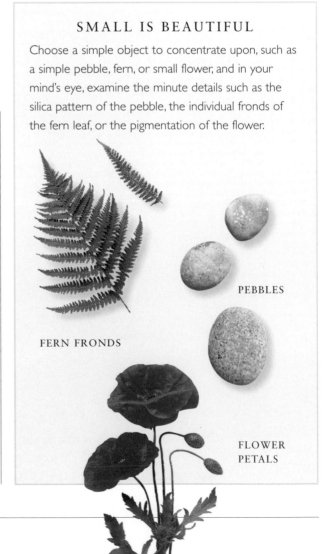

SMALL IS BEAUTIFUL

Choose a simple object to concentrate upon, such as a simple pebble, fern, or small flower, and in your mind's eye, examine the minute details such as the silica pattern of the pebble, the individual fronds of the fern leaf, or the pigmentation of the flower.

PEBBLES

FERN FRONDS

FLOWER PETALS

Heaven and Earth Meditation

This is a "Heaven and Earth meditation," which I often do as a guided visualization. Find a quiet place where you will be undisturbed for five or ten minutes. Get into a comfortable sitting position, then close your eyes and see yourself in your mind's eye in the room where you are. Imagine yourself floating up to the ceiling of the room, and then out through the roof into the air above the building. Very slowly float upward so that you can see the rooftops and trees, then higher and higher until you become aware of the larger geographical features: hills, lakes, and rivers. Continue up higher until you can see the whole country and the ocean lying beneath you. Then become aware of the continents and, as you go even higher, of the Earth as a planet. Finally rest out in space looking back at the green and blue sphere that is our Earth. How far away and precious it looks, shining bright in the immensity of space. You cannot see any wars or disasters or your own troubles, just a beautiful round wholeness.

Now slowly come back down toward the Earth through the atmosphere toward your continent. Gradually descend toward your own country, thinking about how it relates the countries and oceans around it. As you draw nearer to your country, notice the seas, then the hills, rivers, towns, houses, and trees. Back you come to above the building where you began, and down into the room where you are sitting. Take a deep breath, in and out.

Now you are going to imagine yourself feeling very heavy, so heavy that you sink down through the floor into the ground. Slip down into the moist earth and see the roots of plants and trees, the tunnels made by mice and moles, and stones, and maybe old, buried ruins. Down you sink through a layer of rock, coming out into a subterranean cavern with a river running through; glittering and dripping, stalagmites and stalactites decorate its floor and ceiling. Go down even farther and you reach a cave where crystals twinkle. It feels warm and safe here, as if you are held in the arms of the Mother Earth. Now slowly retrace your steps up through the layers of rock, the stones and streams, up through the fertile earth where the roots of plants feed, back up to the light, and into your own room. Bring yourself back into awareness of yourself sitting in your chair, in this time and place. Slowly stretch and move a little, and when you feel quite ready, open your eyes.

That is one of my favorite guided meditations. It gives a sense of perspective and yet connection with the Earth and our place on it. Once you have done it a few times you can actually take yourself on that trip quite swiftly, and, like me, you may find it has a very centering effect in times of stress.

RIGHT *Heaven and Earth meditation gives a sense of our own connection with the earth.*

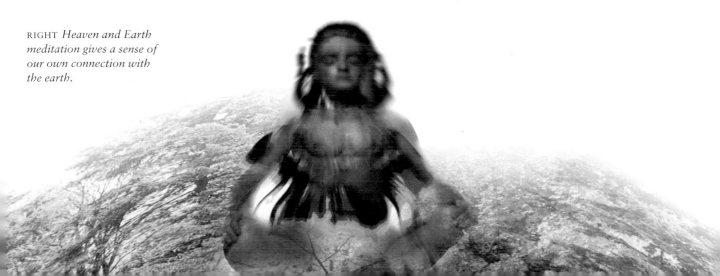

Rainbow Meditation

The following visualization activates the chakras through the use of color and allows you to let go of any problems that may be troubling you.

Lie down flat, somewhere comfortable and draft-free. Close your eyes and relax the muscles of your face, making sure your teeth are not clenched. Imagine that you are in a quiet meadow in the country. It's very warm and peaceful, the sun is shining on your face, and you can hear the sounds of birds calling.

In your mind's eye, see yourself getting up and walking slowly around the meadow. Notice the plants growing along the hedgerow, where there are wild roses, all pink and red; in another corner there are marigolds in different shades of orange and yellow. And the long grass is very green and lush with many types of delicate fronds and seed heads in colors ranging from pale yellowy-green, through warm grass green, to shades of aquamarine. Walk around the fence until you come to a gate. Open the gate and walk down a pathway that leads you to a stream. As you sit down on the soft grass among the waving reeds at the edge of the stream, observe how clear the water is as it chatters over the stones and around the reeds. Notice how flexible it is, flowing around obstacles – sometimes faster, sometimes slower, but always going onward. Watch the deep green underwater plants bending gracefully with the flow of the stream, but never moving from their firm roothold in the river bed.

If you have some worry or unresolved problem, imagine that you are physically carrying it around with you. Take it out of your pocket, and in your mind's eye put it onto a small piece of tree bark you find beside you. Launch it into the water and watch the stream carry it away to be resolved in the course of time when it reaches the ocean.

Now imagine you sit back and let your gaze wander up to the blue sky. It's very clear with only a few little clouds. There's no wind so they hardly move in the upper atmosphere. Look directly above you where the sky is so deep a blue as to be almost purple. Allow your eyes to relax into infinity. Then slowly come back. Bring your gaze back from the blue sky, thinking of yourself standing up slowly, and retrace your steps up the path to the meadow. Go back through the gate and close it. Wander around the meadow noticing the green grass, the yellow and orange marigolds, and the pink and red roses, until you reach the place where you began your journey.

Imagine yourself to be lying down again in your quiet meadow. Take three or four deep, relaxing breaths, and slowly come back to the here and now.

BELOW *Meditating on the colors of nature allows us to let go of troubling problems.*

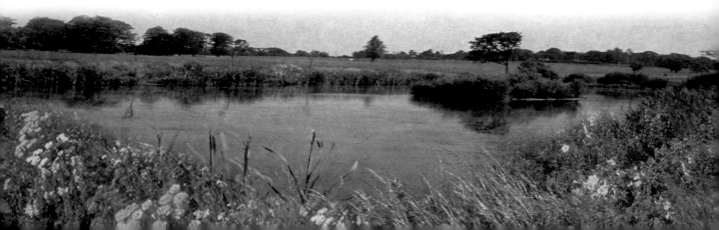

Personal Meditation

This meditation is good if you find it difficult to relax physically.

It is best to lie down in a quiet, comfortable place. Begin by noticing your breathing. Don't try to change it or deepen it, just notice how fast or slowly you are breathing and where the breath is going. Now take your consciousness to your feet. Be aware of all the little bones in your feet, and in your mind's eye imagine all the connections between them relaxing and loosening, so that your feet feel wider and larger. Now imagine your ankle and Achilles tendon. See the tendon lengthening and the ankle becoming more flexible. Think of your calf muscles and allow them to become soft. Now take your consciousness to the big muscles of your thighs, front and back. Notice if they feel tight or are aching; be aware of any of the muscle fibers running along them. Feel the muscle fibers melting and allowing the tension to flow away. Now bring your attention to your hara: let your abdominal muscles relax so that your internal organs can rest comfortably in their proper places. Feel the sensation of everything in your middle flopping down or outward. Let your body feel heavy, as if it is making a deep impression on the mattress beneath you. Let the small of you back go. Notice how good it feels when you don't have to hold anything up any more.

Next take your attention to your spine. Feel it resting on the floor and notice the places where it touches it. Allow the muscles in your buttocks at the base of your spine to melt and relax. In your mind's eye, see the vertebrae and imagine the spaces between them easing out so that you have the sensation of the spine lengthening and loosening, enabling more of it to come into contact with the ground. Take a deep breath into your chest, and as you breathe out, feel your shoulders relaxing onto the floor. Let your arms flop palm upward, feeling so heavy that you can't lift them.

Be aware of your neck and head. Imagine the neck muscles as cords attaching your head to your shoulders. Now see those cords becoming loose, especially the ones at the side of the neck. Feel your scalp melt and your face feel heavy; you can let your mouth fall open and relax your tongue. Remain like this for a little while, then breathe to hara to bring yourself back to the everyday world.

> ### CAUTION
> You could record some of these meditations onto a tape to listen to, but if you do, please do not play them while driving a car.

BELOW *Becoming aware of our own bodies through meditation can aid relaxation.*

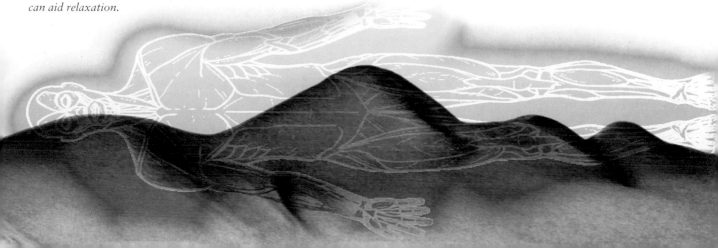

5 Food

"You are what you eat," we are told frequently, and certainly common sense tells us that there is a connection. What most of us are not so aware of are the more subtle energetic effects that food can have on our health, our moods, and our overall state of Ki. There are so many different dietary regimes that we may be forgiven for wondering what is best to eat, and, with pollution, irradiation, and chemicals all part of modern-day living, for asking if it is safe to eat anything at all!

There is no definite answer. The traditional oriental view of diet looks for a balance of the "five flavors" (bitter, sweet, pungent, salty, and sour) from the Five Element correspondences, and a balance of Yin or Yang foods according to the time of year and the needs of the individual. Macrobiotics, which is a modern derivation of traditional Japanese diet, also classifies food and cooking methods by the Yin Yang principle: Yang foods grow below or on the ground, Yin foods above the ground or on bushes and trees. Yang cooking is slower, with pressure or in an oven and with salt; Yin methods include steaming, and raw food. Some people find the guidelines provided by Macrobiotics immensely useful, especially in cases of illness; others find them too restricting. Traditional Chinese Medicine also has a dietary aspect; it classifies foods according to their warming or cooling properties and by the traditional flavors, of each which affects our bodies in a different way.

Personally, I feel that whatever dietary regime you follow, food should be a pleasure, not a source of stress or guilt. Eating meals should be a social activity not something that is snatched, or done furtively, or involves obsessive calorie counting – these are the first steps to eating disorders. We should eat in order to live, not the other way around. Each of us must find our ideal diet and let it work positively for us. There is not space in this book to go into detail about all the factors involved in good nutrition; however, most dietary therapists and nutritionists would agree with the following simple guidelines to ensure good health.

1. Make sure that you eat regularly, chewing your food properly, and don't eat if you are feeling particularly stressed or angry.

2. Eat plenty of fruit and vegetables – ideally organic if you have a source, or homegrown. Two portions of vegetables (either cooked or raw) and at least one piece of fruit per day is a rough guide.

3. Make sure you take enough protein: beans, tofu, fish (not farmed), eggs (free range). If you eat red meat, try to restrict it to once or twice a week. Some people like to eat their protein separately from carbohydrates, since this can ease digestion.

4. Increase your intake of whole grains, such as brown rice, millet, buckwheat, oats, and barley. Sources of fiber are wholemeal pasta, couscous, nuts, and seeds.

5. Many people do not digest bread very well, either because of wheat allergy or the yeast used. Substitute oatcakes, ricecakes, or rye crispbreads.

6. Stimulants such as tea, coffee, chocolate, sugar, and the chemicals found in processed and packaged food are in general not beneficial for our health. Herb teas, coffee substitutes, pure fruit juices, and plain spring water are the best drinks, but if you are very attached to your stimulating caffeine try to have just one or two cups per day. Sugar can be just as addictive; use honey instead. In

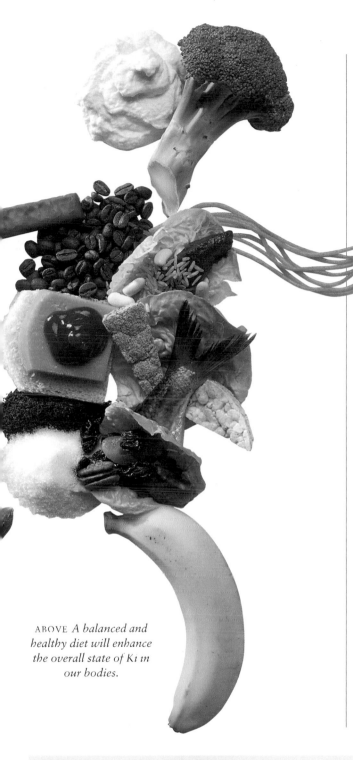

ABOVE *A balanced and healthy diet will enhance the overall state of Ki in our bodies.*

the long run, giving up sugar could well be the most beneficial, health-promoting measure you could make in your diet.

7. Some people have problems digesting dairy products, because they can lead to an overproduction of mucus, resulting in sinus trouble, and digestive and skin complaints. Children are often sensitive to milk, and in cases of eczema and asthma, you could try cutting out milk for a couple of months, as this may help considerably but check with your physician first. Soy milk and tofu (soybean) products, which are more acceptable to sensitive digestions, are now available in health food stores and many supermarkets.

8. If you snack between meals, try to go for fruit, dried fruit, nuts, or raw vegetables rather than candy or cakes. Some people need to work on the "little-and-often" principle, especially if they have a tendency to blood-sugar swings. In this case, a handful of almonds, sunflower seeds, and raisins can be just as satisfying and, in the long run, better for health.

9. Finally, make sure that you drink a glass or two of plain water every day. The body needs a certain amount of water in order to carry on its necessary chemical processes; dehydration can result if this is not supplied. Water also helps to flush out toxins and cleanse the body.

CHANGING YOUR DIET SENSIBLY

If you are changing your diet, it is a good idea to introduce new measures slowly. There will be less chance of digestive problems or the family staging a mutiny when their favorite junk food is taken off the menu! I find that a wholefood, vegetarian diet suits my system best, since it provides plenty of energy and variety. As a Shiatsu practitioner I have a few personal rules, like not taking alcohol or very sweet food on days when I am practicing or teaching. On the other hand, I find that it does no harm to stray from the straight and narrow occasionally. There is nothing worse than people whose diet is so restricted (by choice, not for medical reasons, I might add) that you can't take them out for dinner!

6 Lifestyle

Two other factors in good health that must not be forgotten are exercise and sleep. However fast a pace we live at, or whatever our lifestyle, sleep and exercise are essential. Two categories of exercise are relevant here: aerobic exercise that increases the heart-rate and speeds up circulation, such as running, cycling, swimming, team games, racquet sports, and even a brisk walk; and soft exercise that improves Ki circulation and flexibility, such as yoga, Tai Chi, Qi Gong, Do-In, and so on. I would suggest that everyone should do a little of each; 20 minutes' brisk exercise to stimulate the cardiovascular system three times per week and 15 minutes' soft exercise every day are good averages to aim for.

Sleep and rest are just as important. During the night our bodies rest and recuperate, building up our store of Ki for use the next day. Either too much sleep or too little can have a detrimental effect, but each of us must discover what routine works best for us and try to be reasonably consistent. The gentle movements we make during sleeping hours allow us to relax and unknot our bodies subconsciously, while dreams may help us to work through the unfinished affairs of the day.

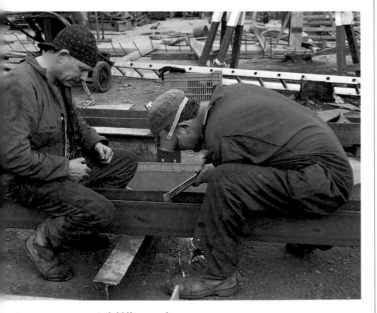

ABOVE *A fulfilling and responsible occupation is one of the most important ways of giving life a purpose.*

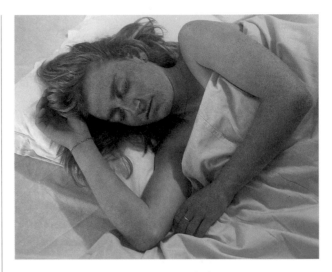

ABOVE *Getting enough sleep in a comfortable, supportive bed in a well-ventilated bedroom helps to replenish the store of Ki.*

Insomnia is a problem for many people, and in my experience it is the worry about not sleeping that is often more of a problem than the lack of sleep itself. If you find you wake up at night and cannot get off to sleep again, don't worry. Although our bodies need sleep, they need rest just as much – tell yourself that although you are not sleeping, you are resting, and try some of the hara breathing exercises we looked at earlier in this section. After ten minutes or so of these, you may find that your mind has quieted sufficiently to let you nod off again.

FINDING A SENSE OF PURPOSE

Perhaps the most important aspect of lifestyle for everybody is to have a job, area of activity, or hobby that gives a sense of purpose in life. Most of us at some stage in our lives ask ourselves the questions "What is the point of all this?" or "Why am I here?" Having some sphere of activity that puts life into perspective and gives it meaning is essential for our long-term spiritual and mental happiness. This, of course, varies vastly according to each of us. The doctor performing a difficult operation, the sleep-deprived parents with an overactive child, the sports instructor still on the field teaching with a broken collarbone, or the musician entertaining a packed

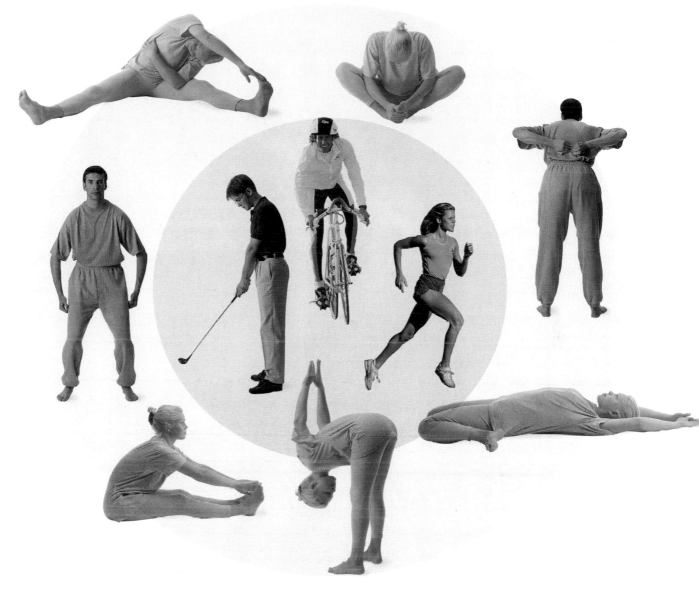

ABOVE *A balance of aerobic exercise such as cycling, running, or golf, and gentler forms such as yoga or Shiatsu Makko-ho stretches, help maintain fitness and flexibility.*

concert hall – all have a motivation that gives purpose and structure to their lives.

Another aspect of lifestyle which is frequently neglected in our fast-moving society is that of "being" not "doing." It is important to "do" the right things: exercise, eat good food, engage in supportive activities. But it is equally important to spend time by yourself just "being" – without any pressure to achieve, act, or "do" in any way.

That might sound selfish, but in truth, the time you spend nurturing yourself in this way is the foundation from which you can go out into the world knowing who you are and what you want. Moreover, if you are not so positive about where you're going, at least the peace that you gain from a little self reflection can help to set you on the road.

So often in my practice I see people who have come to Shiatsu for physical reasons – for a bad back, or a migraine – but behind the pain there is a feeling of being at a crossroads, of not being certain of their direction. The Ki centering and grounding exercises and the self-help measures we have discussed here can help to put them sufficiently in touch with themselves to begin to find their sense of purpose.

7 First Aid Points

Although a relaxing Shiatsu session may be just what we need when we are ill or in pain, sometimes it is not practical. This is where we can make use of specific tsubo for first aid. Each practitioner has a list of useful points, and those below are the ones if I find most helpful in situations where a full session is not possible. Where you are using a tsubo as a remedy for a specific complaint, do remember that it is not a "magic bullet," and results may not be immediate. For example, if I use a point for a headache, I usually find that it takes about 15 minutes of working the point on and off to produce a reduction in the pain.

Press the point and get the sensation of connecting with Ki – generally a "nice pain" or sensitivity. Hold that for between 7 and 10 seconds, then release for the same length of time. Continue on and off for a couple of minutes and then rest for a couple of minutes. If the point starts to feel very sensitive, try using another point with a similar action – points can often be used very effectively in combinations.

BELOW *The position of the main "First Aid" points, shown in detail on the following pages.*

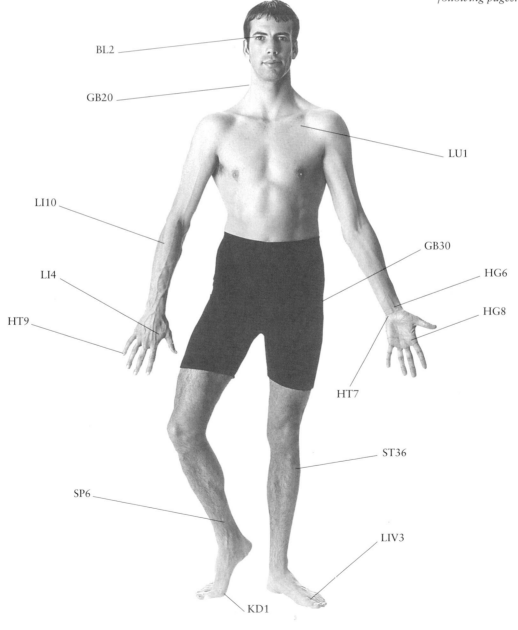

BL 2

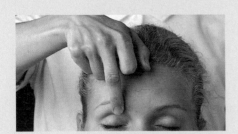

BL2: *in the notch at the inside of the upper eye socket: frontal headache and sore eyes.*

LI 10

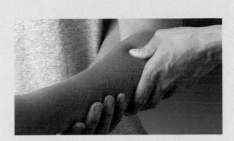

LI10: *three fingers' width down from the elbow crease, on top of the large forearm muscle: this helps in pain control in the arm and shoulders, intestinal problems.*

GB 20

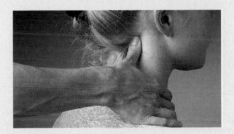

GB20: *on the hollow between the two large neck muscles (trapezius and sternocleidomastoid) at the back of the neck, just under the skull: this is the neck release point for tension and pain in the neck, or one-sided headaches.*

LU 1

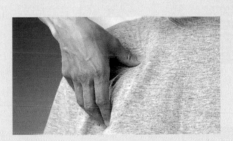

LU1: *one thumb's width below the hollow under the outside end of the collarbone: coughing, asthma, any lung problem.*

HG 6

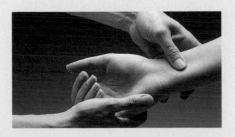

HG6: *two thumbs' width above the wrist crease on the inner arm, between the tendons: useful to control nausea and vomiting, especially morning sickness and travel sickness.*

LI 4

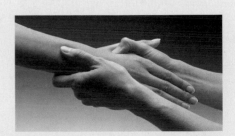

LI4: *in the fleshy web between thumb and index finger close to the bones: headaches, toothaches, constipation, diarrhea, general toning of the intestines, helps to promote labor but otherwise forbidden in pregnancy.*

HG 8

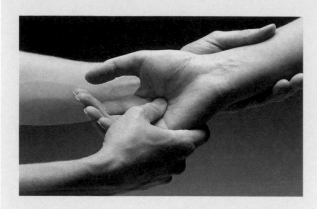

HG8: *if you make a loose fist, HG8 is where your middle finger touches the center of your palm, between the bones that join the index and middle fingers. This tsubo is useful for calming the mind if you are nervous or anxious. Its oriental name is "The Palace of Weariness," sometimes translated as "Palace of Labor." It is particularly effective for certain Heat conditions that involve fever and mental symptoms.*

HT 7

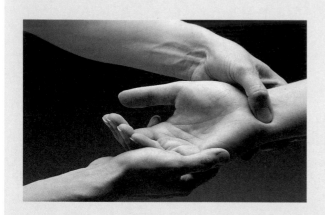

HT7: *at the wrist crease in line with the inside of the little finger is the "corner" formed by the prominent pisiform bone on the hand and the flexor tendon that attaches to it. This is one of the most important tsubo in the body. Its action is principally to calm the mind in cases of anxiety, stress, worry, and mental disturbance. In addition it can be used for palpitations, poor memory, and insomnia, all of which are symptoms of imbalance. in the Heart energy.*

HT 9

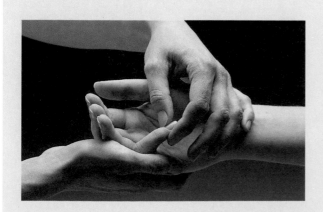

HT9: *on the inside corner of the fingernail at the nail bed. This point can be used for heart problems including heart attack (if other first aid measures have been taken), and a sensation of fullness and stuffiness in the heart area. Emotionally it is good for excessive symptoms such as hysteria or serious anxiety. traditionally HT9 has also been used in cases of unconsciousness.*

GB30

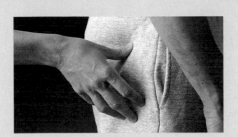

GB30: *in the center of the buttock where there is a hollow when the muscle is clenched: sciatica, pain, and tiredness in the legs, lower back pain.*

ST36

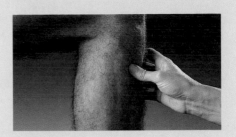

ST36: *with the knee bent, three thumbs' width below the hollow at the outside bottom corner of the kneecap, and one finger's width out from the crest of the anterior tibial muscle: any stomach disorder, tiredness and pain in the legs, good for vitality.*

SP6

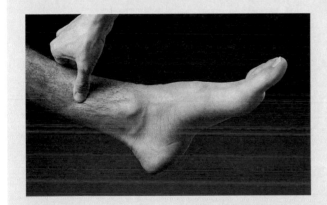

SP6: *four fingers' width up from the highest part of the inner ankle, just behind the tibia bone: this can help with menstrual problems of any sort, especially menstrual pain, reproductive disorders, tiredness, relieves pain in the abdomen, calms the mind, insomnia. Avoid during pregnancy, but useful in labor.*

LIV3

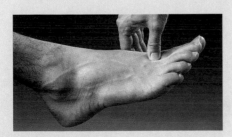

LIV3: *on the top of the foot in the hollow behind the second joint of the big toe, between first and second metatarsals: this point helps with migraines, headaches, muscular cramps, calming effect, especially on bad temper.*

KD1

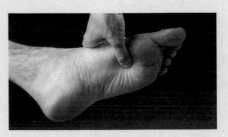

KD1: *on the sole of the foot just below the ball, in line with the second toe: tonifies the body's Yin energy, clears and calms the mind, can be used in cases of unconsciousness.*

8 Moxibustion

Moxibustion is often used by Shiatsu practitioners in combination with Shiatsu to promote healing in cases where heat is beneficial. Processed from the common herb mugwort, moxa is burned either on or above specific tsubo in order to warm them, encourage local circulation, and deliberately increase Ki flow into a particular point.

Moxa punk looks a bit like brown absorbent cotton. When used with the "direct" method, it is pinched into little cones, which are then burned down on a thin slice of ginger or garlic until the receiver feels a hot sensation.

Rather more practical and less difficult to use during a Shiatsu session is the "indirect" method, where the moxa punk has been compressed into a roll, like a long cigar, and this is held over the point, on and off, until it becomes reddish and feels pleasantly warm.

Since moxa does not burn with a flame but merely smolders, it is quite easy to regulate the heat by holding it closer or farther away, and the receiver is instructed to say when it becomes too hot. It goes without saying that the practitioner takes great care not to burn the skin.

Treatment by moxa is very effective for cases of chronic pain, frozen shoulder, some kinds of arthritis, diarrhea, coldness, and general tiredness.

ACHIEVING CONTROL

All of the adjuncts to treatment and exercises described in this section can be incorporated into our everyday lives when we start to take more responsibility for ourselves. By doing them we can feel and understand that by our own actions, activities, and attitudes, we can change our Ki state to one where we can become more in control of ourselves and better able to achieve what we want to in life.

EQUIPMENT FOR MOXIBUSTION

The equipment needed for direct moxibustion comprises moxa punk (as shown below) either hand rolled into appropriate sized cones, or preformed cones, plus thin slices of ginger or garlic. The indirect method, more popular with Shiatsu practitioners, requires only a moxa stick, an ashtray, and either a special snuffer or a bowl of sand to extinguish the stick at the end of the treatment.

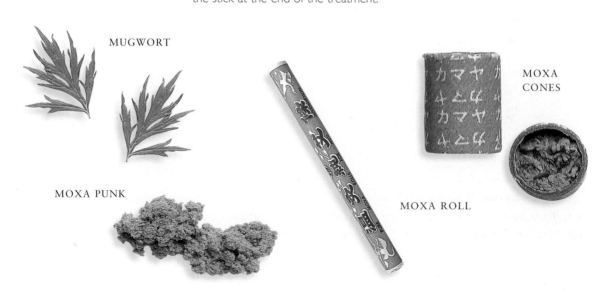

MUGWORT

MOXA PUNK

MOXA ROLL

MOXA CONES

INDIRECT MOXIBUSTION

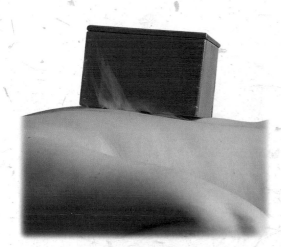

A moxa box, such as this one, can be used to heat up a large area and is therefore helpful if several adjacent tsubo are need to be heated. It is a more general warming method than heating specific points.

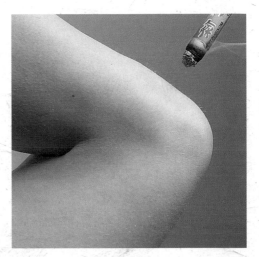

This is the method most usually practiced by Shiatsu therapists. The moxa stick is held over a point with a particular therapeutic benefit. The stick is applied for several minutes until the point becomes red or until the patient lets the practitioner know the heat is too much.

DIRECT MOXIBUSTION

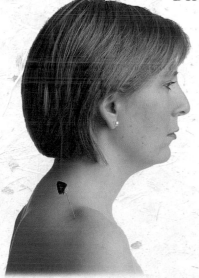

Acupuncturists use the direct method of moxibustion more frequently than Shiatsu practitioners. In this case, the moxa cone is held in a special cup and the heat is transmitted into the body through the needle.

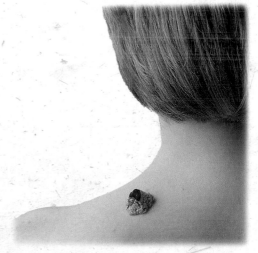

Direct moxa can be "scarring" or "non-scarring." The non-scarring method is generally used for cosmetic reasons and the moxa cone is placed on a slice of ginger. Here a very large cone is being burnt, but would be removed before scarring occurred.

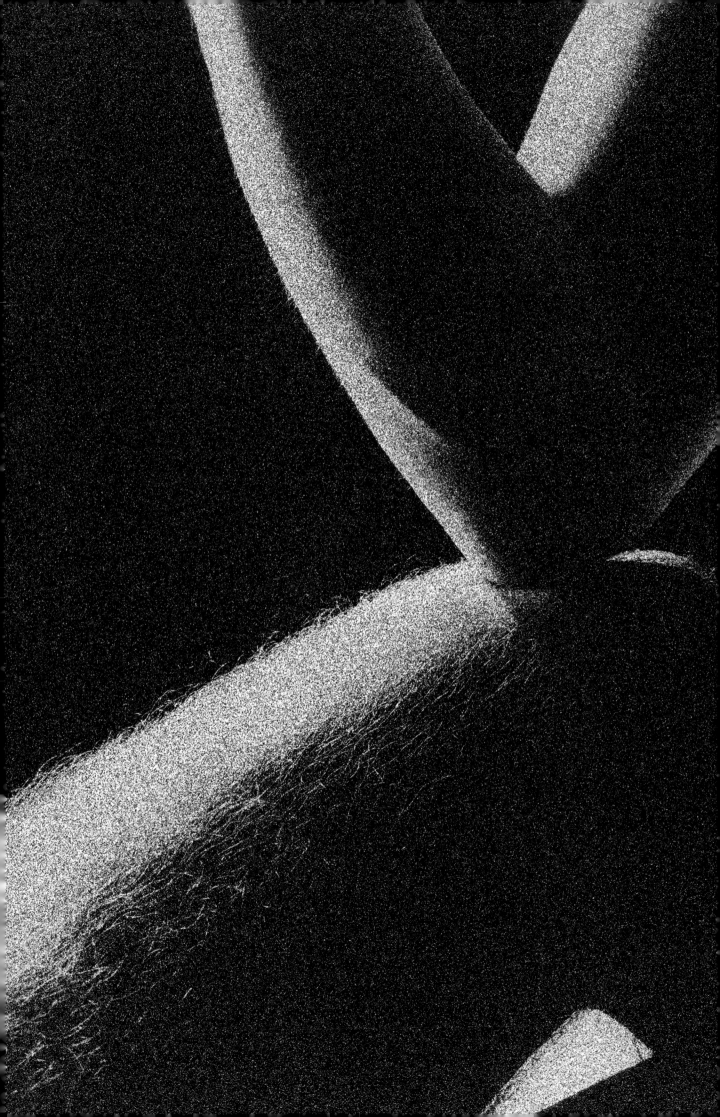

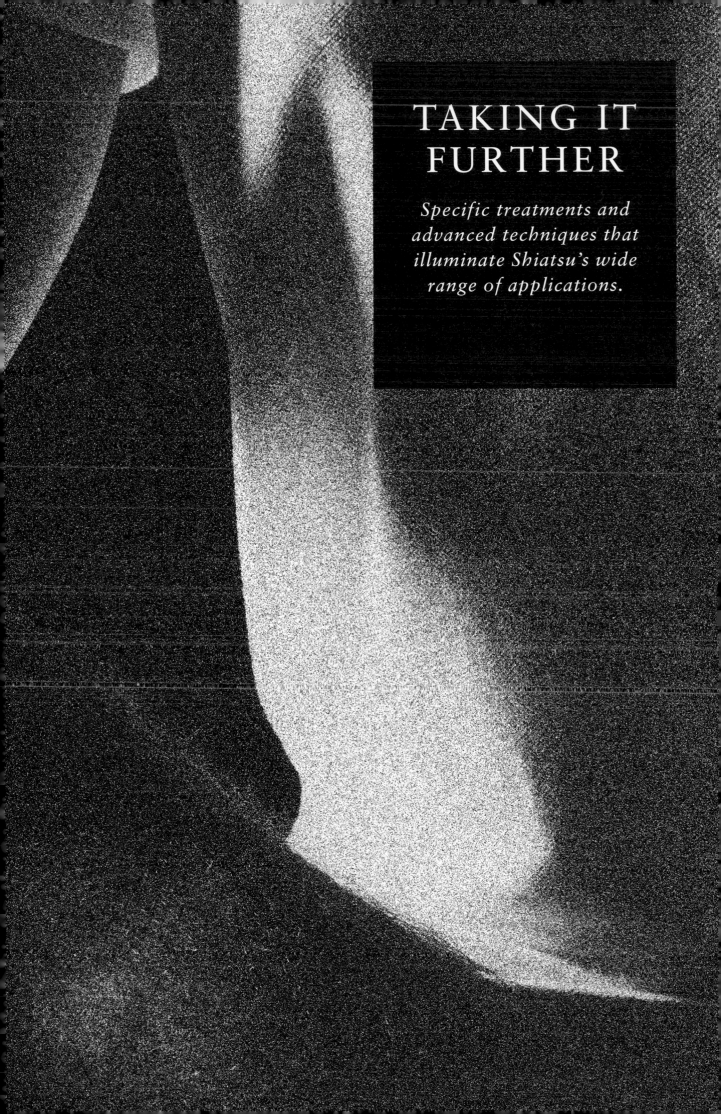

TAKING IT FURTHER

Specific treatments and advanced techniques that illuminate Shiatsu's wide range of applications.

1 Low Back Pain

Back pain accounts for a large proportion of many Shiatsu practitioners' work. Although pain or imbalance can have energy-related causes on several levels, it is often most useful to explain back pain in terms of the physical: the muscular and/or bone dysfunction.

Back pain caused by a slipped disk is actually relatively rare. What is usually causing the pain is spasm of the deep and postural muscles in and around the back, or, in the case of lower backache, a displacement of the sacroiliac joint.

In my practice, if someone turns up with back pain, having initially done a hara diagnosis, I will check out the sacroiliac joint, and if this is compromised I will do a simple adjustment to restore the joint to correct alignment. Next, I will check out the Yu points in the back. Very often a lordosis, or excessive inward curve of the lumbar area, will denote imbalance in the Kidney or Large Intestine meridians. The lordosis may also be a sign of tightness or spasm in the iliopsoas muscle. In my own experience, disturbance in psoas is a major cause of lower back pain, as well as sciatica. A third area of inquiry would be tightness in the piriformis muscle, which runs in the buttock, and which can cause diverse symptoms ranging from persistent pain in the lower back and hips, to sciatica, rotation of the pelvis, and even to shortening of the leg on the affected side.

Sometimes, as someone lies down, you will notice the muscles on one side of the spine are more prominent than on the other. This is usually due to long-term holding on in the deep muscles that run all the way up the back. Working the Bladder meridian throughout the length of the back in a slow and deep way allows these muscles to release and even out.

Many of the classical acupuncture points for back pain are in fact known to Western science as trigger points, which generate referred pain in specific locations elsewhere in the body, and this phenomenon can be used to good effect by removing the tightness in the muscles that is the cause of the problem.

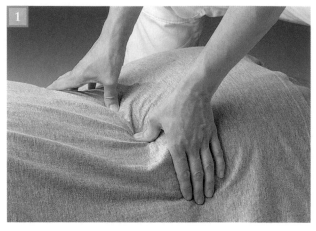

One thumb is working on the Large Intestine Yu point (BL25, located between the fourth and fifth lumbar vertebrae), while the other finds trigger points, or Ahshi points, along the top of the iliac crest.

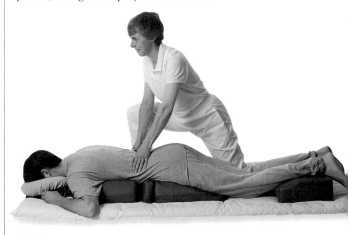

2 *It is usually a good idea to pad up your partner if his or her back is painful, in order not to accentuate the lumbar curve by lying flat. Pillows can be used as easily as the special support shown here.*

When treating someone specifically for back pain there is no set routine. I have described earlier my general line of enquiry to try and find out the physical cause of the problem. Having come to a conclusion, I would use my hara diagnosis as a basis for working intuitively on the back, making use of diagnostic areas, Yu points, areas where I know from experience that tension or weakness may occur. Many points are known to assist in the relief of back pain, and they can all be worked gently with the thumbs or fingers, or, if appropriate, can be stimulated deeply with the elbows. Many of these points are best used in combination with a strong mother hand. Examples of effective techniques are shown on the next few pages.

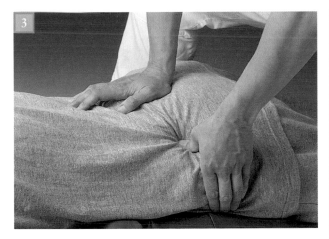

A hand on the sacrum feels very supportive and nurturing in cases of chronic, or long-term, back pain. To thumb the piriformis muscle that runs deep in the buttock, work a line from the sacrum to the top of the femur.

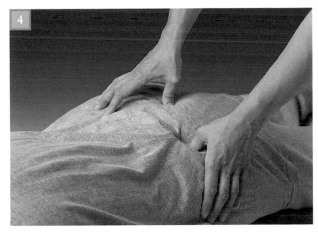

The origin of the piriformis is along the edge of the sacroiliac joint. Sensitive pressure here can help both to release the muscle and to stimulate the supplementary Kidney meridian, which is often involved in back pain.

CAUTION

It is sometimes better to wait 24 hours in cases of severe back pain to let the Ki settle in the area before working on it.

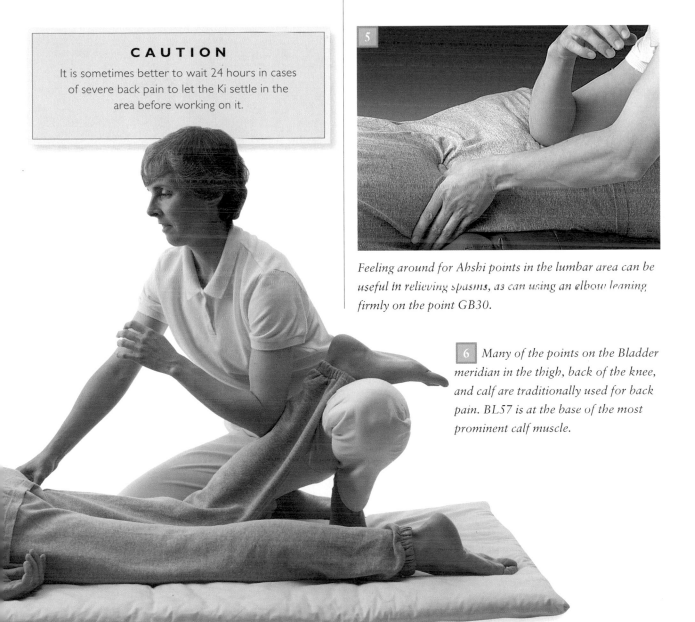

Feeling around for Ahshi points in the lumbar area can be useful in relieving spasms, as can using an elbow leaning firmly on the point GB30.

6 Many of the points on the Bladder meridian in the thigh, back of the knee, and calf are traditionally used for back pain. BL57 is at the base of the most prominent calf muscle.

Back Pain 2

Working in the side position can be very helpful where your partner has difficulty lying on his or her back or front. Frequently in this position the deep back muscles will relax spontaneously and allow greater access to the Bladder meridian to balance out the energies. Also, the Gall Bladder meridian in the buttock and side of leg can be easily worked like this. Have your partner comfortably padded up with pillows under the head and top side leg, so that he or she doesn't topple over.

The supine position is also very useful for back problems, as we saw in the Basic Sequence and the case histories. Remember that leg rotations loosen up the pelvic area, including the buttocks. The Kidney stretch, pushing one knee toward the opposite shoulder (see step 26 of the Basic Sequence) is particularly helpful in stretching the piriformis and can be used as a self-help measure very easily. In addition, working the Stomach meridian in the groin area can assist in loosening up the insertion of the iliopsoas muscle.

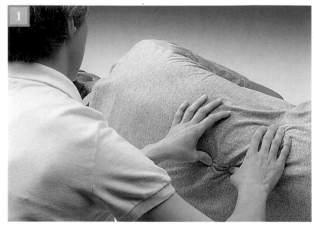

Use two thumbs on the same side of the spine to work intuitively on parts of the Bladder meridian that feel imbalanced.

CAUTION

In cases of back pain, always work gently and generally to begin with. Specific thumb techniques can be used once you have gauged the level of energetic and muscular holding, and the receiver's pain threshold.

palm pressure is supportive

elbow and knee stretch and support

2 *The palms of the hands can be soothing and relaxing when there is a lot of pain. If pressure is too sore, you can just extend Ki through your palms.*

head padded to keep neck straight

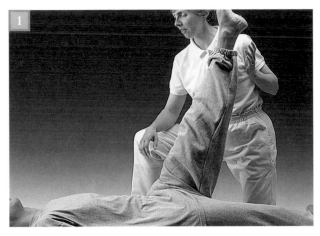

Have your partner breathe in while he or she lifts their leg up straight. Have your thumb resting lightly on ST27, but do not press in yet.

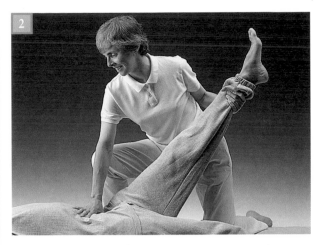

Once the leg is lifted as high as possible, take all the weight of the leg and slowly take it toward the floor as your partner breathes out. At the same time, press into ST27 as far as your partner will allow you.

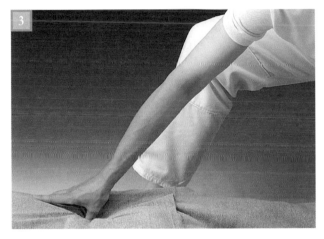

Support the leg all the way down to the floor. Keep the pressure on ST27 and repeat the exercise twice more. You will find that you go deeper into the hara each time. Hold the depth of pressure you have achieved for about 20 seconds at the end of the exercise, and then release slowly.

HARA MASSAGE FOR BACK PAIN

One very effective technique to deal with grumbling pain caused by spasm in the psoas muscle is shown here. Because the fibers of the iliopsoas originate on the front surfaces of the lumbar vertebrae and the inside of the ilium and sacrum, and run through the pelvis to insert on the inside of the top of the femur, the only way actually to touch the main part of the muscle is to work deep into the hara. Begin by finding point ST27, two cun out and down from the navel. Steps 1 to 3 talk you through the technique, but it is important to keep the deep pressure on without releasing it to make the exercise effective. It may feel as if you are pressing right through your partner's intestines to the spine – well, you should be to do this properly, so be brave!

This exercise can be incorporated into an ordinary Shiatsu sequence at any point when you are working on the front of the legs.

padding to
support knee

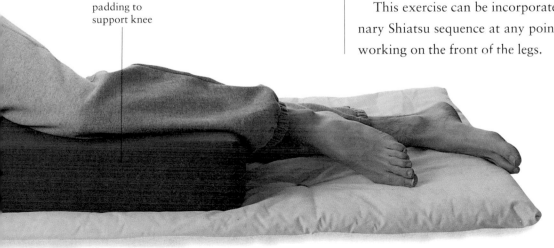

2 Menstrual Problems

Menstrual complaints commonly react well to Shiatsu treatment. The meridians involved may be Spleen, Liver, or Kidney (the three Yin meridians that run in the leg), which may be affected by excesses or deficiencies. For example, one of the functions of the Spleen is to "control the Blood." If it is too weak to do so, excessive bleeding may result. Likewise, if the Liver meridian is stagnant, it will be unable to fulfill its function of regulating the movement of Ki and blood around the body, with the result that periods may be painful. The Kidney's essential function is to store our Jing, which governs birth, growth, and reproduction. Overwork, stress, irregular meals, and an imbalance between mental work and physical activity can deplete our Yin forces and our Jing, which can lead to infertility and (in combination with Liver deficiency), and an associated lack of periods.

In Five Element terms, we can sum up the functions of these different meridians by saying that Earth (Spleen) is responsible for the cycles and for ensuring that the "soil" of the body, the uterus, is ripe for receiving the seed. Water (Kidneys) provides the motivation, desire, and ability to reproduce, while Wood (Liver) is in charge of the actual movement of Ki that allows reproduction to take place (that is, the sexual act, erection, and ejaculation in men, and the movement of Ki involved in the menstrual cycle for women).

To categorize all the different syndromes and symptoms that may present themselves in relation to menstrual disturbances is beyond the scope of this book; however, there are certain points that are extremely helpful to use in combination with steps 31 to 34 of the Basic Sequence. In addition, some general work on the sacrum and lower back can do much to help relieve the backache and cramping that often accompany such periods so you should look again at pages 170-1.

As a general rule, keeping warm is important, especially the hara and the area around the ankles. I am always amazed that people go out in cold weather with insufficient layers of clothing on and without socks or pantyhose. Keeping warm is good for our Ki, and being cold depletes it, meaning that we use much of our precious energy in keeping warm rather than for other essential activities, such as digestion or reproduction.

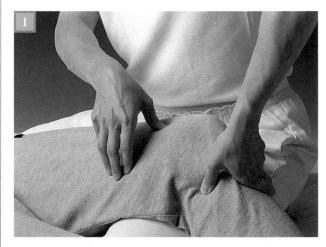

SP9 and SP10: below and above the knee can both feel quite tender and care should be taken when going into these tsubo.

HARA MASSAGE DURING MENSTRUATION

Gentle hara massage can sometimes feel good during your period, and certainly regular work on the hara throughout the month can help the elimination process work more effectively during menstruation. This is something you can do for yourself using the method that is described in the section on Do-in (self-Shiatsu) on page 147.

CAUTION

Do not use SP6 at all during pregnancy, nor apply heavy pressure around the ankles in the first three months. Make sure you check whether your receiver is pregnant first.

2 *The Spleen meridian often needs to be tonified or stimulated along the whole length of the leg. SP6 is a major point to be worked in all menstrual and reproductive imbalances.*

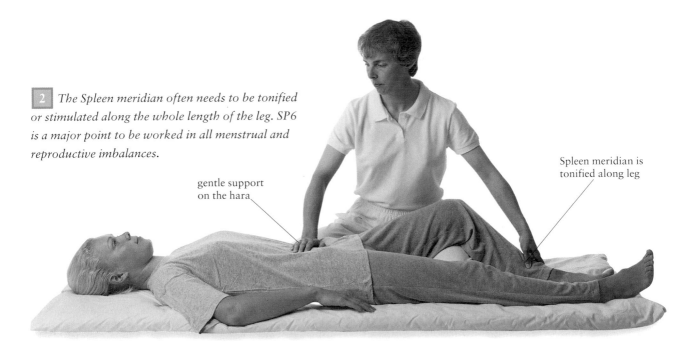

gentle support on the hara

Spleen meridian is tonified along leg

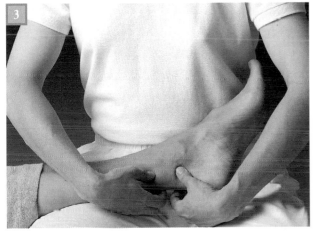

KD3 and KD7 have similar properties in that both nourish and tonify the Kidneys. In working KD3, be sure that your pressure is applied at 90 degrees.

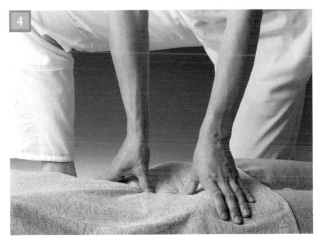

CV4 and CV6 on the midline through the hara can be worked singly or together. Be aware that deep pressure may be uncomfortable if your partner is menstruating.

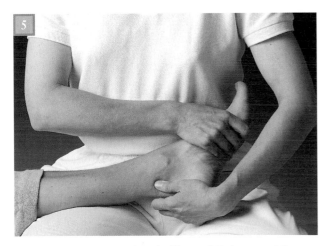

General squeezing on the Bladder and Kidney meridians may feel comforting.

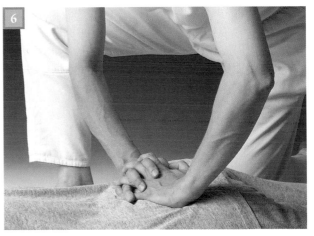

Specific pressure on tender points on the sacrum can do much to relieve the back and abdominal aches that often accompany menstruation.

③ Pregnancy

The purpose of Shiatsu during pregnancy is to promote relaxation and the smooth flow of Ki in the mother-to-be. This is not an appropriate time to be addressing long-term imbalances. Specific treatments should be limited to pregnancy-related conditions such as sciatic pain, tired legs, heartburn, and morning sickness. During the later stages of pregnancy, the emphasis is on preparing the mother's Ki for birth, and, if necessary, helping to ensure the baby is in the correct head-down position.

All the meridians may be affected by pregnancy, but Spleen and Kidney are especially involved: spleen because it is responsible for nourishing the body and helping the development of the fetus, and Kidney because it is the seat of the Jing, the basic vitality and reproductive essence. Both SP and KD can be depleted by pregnancy. Having regular Shiatsu can ensure that energy levels are maintained and potentially serious imbalances do not occur.

Side or sitting positions are the most appropriate to use once the "bump" is showing and it becomes uncomfortable to lie either on the back or face down. Make sure you have plenty of cushions to provide padding under the knee and neck.

One of the major complaints of pregnant women is lower back pain. There may be several different causes of this – sometimes occurring simultaneously. Relaxation of the ligaments in the pelvis may cause problems with the sacroiliac joint, while alteration of the posture due to the extra weight in front is another cause of back pain. Look back to the section on back pain for some useful techniques. Morning sickness, or just not wanting to eat, can be a source of discomfort early on. HG6 is very effective in the treatment of any sort of nausea or vomiting and has been the subject of controlled trials at major hospitals. In the East, acupuncture or moxibustion are traditionally used for turning a breech baby. Applying moxa to BL67 (on the outside end of the little toe, just at the nail bed) has the effect of increasing fetal activity and encouraging the baby to turn head downward.

MERIDIAN

In a general session during pregnancy, the most important meridians to work are Spleen, Kidney, Bladder, and Gall Bladder. All can be reached from a side position, or from a sitting position, although the latter is not as relaxing for a full treatment. As mentioned earlier, Spleen has the function of nourishing both mother and growing baby, while Kidney is where our essential vitality and reproductive potential is stored. Bladder and Gall Bladder are affected symptomatically by pregnancy, in that aches and pains often appear along their pathways, and therefore gentle stimulation can help to ease out any tensions and tiredness in them.

CAUTION

Don't give Shiatsu during the first three months of the pregnancy if there is a history of miscarriage or difficulty in conceiving. For all pregnant women, stimulation below the knee should be avoided; after that, gentle work on ankles and feet is fine. Points SP6, LI4, and GB21 should not be worked at any time, since they all work strongly to bring energy downward in the body and might thus initiate labor.

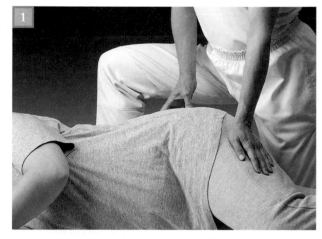

GB30 *in the center of the buttock is effective in easing sciatic pain, but it may be tender to work on, so be sensitive.*

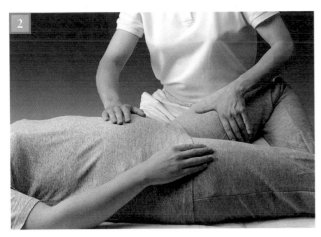

Working with palms, elbows, or "dragon's mouth" on the SP meridian in the thigh has a nurturing effect.

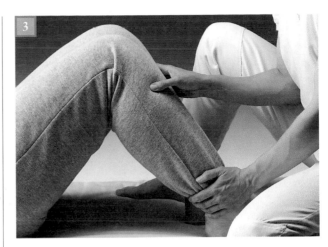

ST36, "Leg Three Miles," is the best point for resolving both heartburn and tired legs. Lying with the knees up is also good for the lower back.

5 *Stimulation of HG6 is helpful in cases of morning sickness. Pressure can be applied by a partner or practitioner, or the pregnant woman can work it herself whenever it is needed. It can be stimulated by means of wrist bands (readily available at a pharmacy for treating travel sickness) or therapeutic magnets that can be stuck on.*

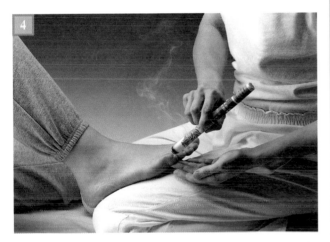

The indirect method of burning moxa, or applying specific pressure on BL67, is traditionally used for turning a breech baby.

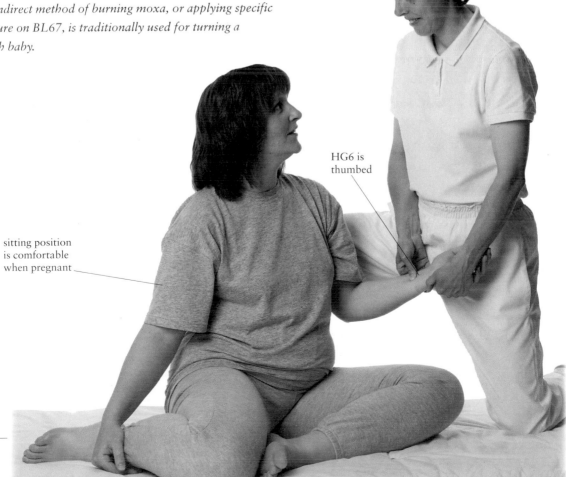

HG6 is
thumbed

sitting position
is comfortable
when pregnant

④ Childbirth

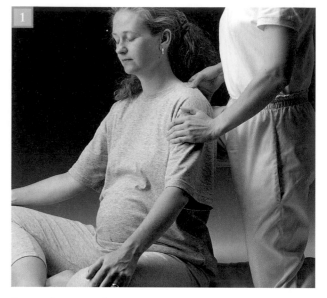

Once the due date for birth has arrived, the quality of Shiatsu can change a little. While the emphasis is still on relaxation and relieving any pains like backache, the tsubo that were previously proscribed can be used to start the birth process. Babies have a habit of arriving in their own good time, when their energy and that of the mother are ripe for labor. So because the action of points is entirely natural and works in harmony with the body's energies, using these specific tsubo is quite safe and will prepare for childbirth.

Having someone to give Shiatsu during labor can be very supportive. These days the birth partner is often taught relaxation and massage techniques to help the process: adding Shiatsu points can assist with pain relief and keep contractions going strongly. However, instances have also been reported where having too much bodywork during labor was distracting and actually slowed things down; also at later stages the mother may become too sensitive to be worked on.

Tiredness, in particular tired legs, is a common complaint during labor. Working generally on Stomach and Bladder meridians can help, and, since both these meridians sustain the downward movement of Ki, can increase contractions. You may find it more useful to work these meridians between contractions than during them.

The treatment position you use during labor will obviously depend on the comfort of the mother. All the techniques described can be performed sitting up, leaning over a beanbag, squatting, or on all fours, or in side lying position. This is a time when you need to be very flexible and creative.

In the postnatal period, the most crucial thing is rest. Regular Shiatsu can help to prevent post-natal depression and establish lactation and the Spleen, Stomach, and Kidney meridians particularly need to be built up for this.

Strong downward pressure on GB21 stimulates hormones that initiate labor and later promote the let-down of milk when the mother is breast feeding.

② *Working on the hollows in the sacrum either with the thumbs or palms is supportive and helps with pain relief. This can be done sitting on a chair, on a beanbag, or lying down.*

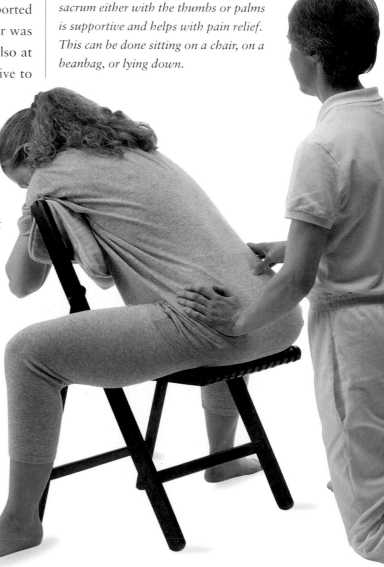

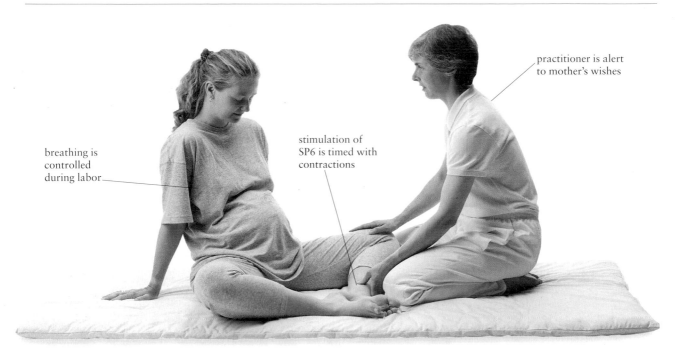

breathing is controlled during labor

stimulation of SP6 is timed with contractions

practitioner is alert to mother's wishes

3 *Points such as SP6 should be used in conjunction with breathing techniques learned at prenatal classes, and the work on them timed to coincide with contractions.*

MERIDIAN

The classic points to set labor going are GB21, LI4, and SP6. These all have the effect of bringing energy downward in the body and thus assisting the baby's Ki to descend. GB21, in particular, has the effect of stimulating the activity of the uterus, so can be used to initiate and strengthen contractions. By the same token, it can help to expel the placenta in the third stage of labor.

SP6 and LI4 can be used to help establish regular contractions and are helpful for pain relief. I personally found SP6 very effective in the first stage of my first labor. ST36 and BL60 can also be used. A graduate from my Shiatsu school recently reported using these during the birth of his son, and said that little other analgesia was required. One of my colleagues had a baby on the day before I wrote this section. They found that pressure on the sacrum and the lumbar area was particularly good for achieving pain relief, the most effective point changing throughout the labor.

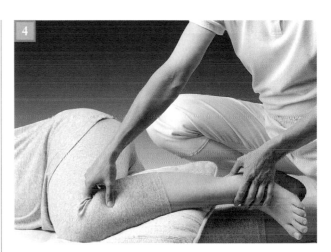

ST36 and BL60 are effective for pain relief. ST36 is particularly helpful for tired and sore legs.

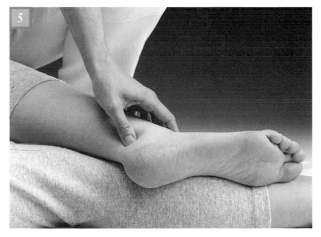

BL60 is located just behind the outer ankle. Deep pressure on this point during contractions is good for controlling pain.

5 Migraine and Headache

Headaches and migraines respond well to Shiatsu, usually in conjunction with lifestyle or dietary changes. Sometimes severe headaches are called migraines, but there is a definite difference between them, to which anyone who has suffered from migraines can testify.

Migraines almost always have a digestive component to them in that the sufferer may feel nauseous or actually vomit. Digestion usually stops, which is why medication often has little or no effect, since it is taken too late. The sufferer may experience sensitivity to light or noise, and classically there is visual disturbance before the head pain starts. Even severe, debilitating headaches do not have these features.

Locating the seat of the headache is an important factor in determining the cause and, to a certain extent, in choosing appropriate treatment. Headaches and migraines may have similar causes and are often treated in a similar way. Stress and tight musculature in the neck and shoulders is often a contributory factor. Trigger points develop in certain neck muscles, particularly the sternocleidomastoid, and these can refer pain up into the head. A very common pain pattern is the one-sided headache,

MERIDIAN

The main meridians to treat in all cases of headaches are Bladder and Gall Bladder. In addition to the specific points and techniques illustrated, GB20 and LI4 are powerful tsubo for pain relief and dispersing excessive Ki. The former is particularly good for headaches located at the side or back of the head, and for stiff neck. Stress and overwork can deplete Spleen Ki and in the long term, Kidney Ki. Anger, frustration, and irritability affect the Liver meridian, whose energy then rises up and gets stuck in the head. Also trigger foods can affect migraine sufferers, and food sensitivities of this sort may involve Stomach, Spleen, Liver, and Kidney meridians.

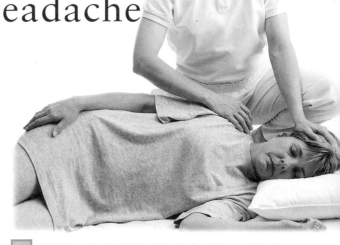

1 Working the Gall Bladder in the side position is a comfortable way of getting into useful points on the head and neck that are effective for headaches.

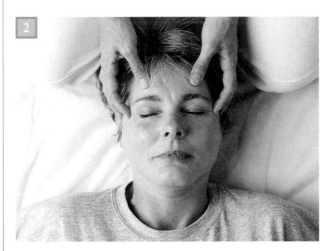

GB1, at the outside corner of the eye, and GB14, midway up the forehead in line with the pupil, are often the focus of pain. Gentle stimulation can disperse tension.

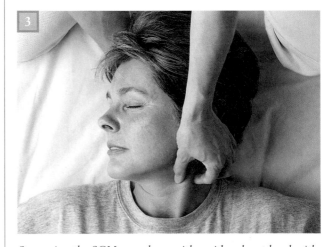

Squeezing the SCM muscle on either side, about level with the Adam's apple, taps into LI18 and ST9; both are sites of trigger points that refer pain to the side of the head.

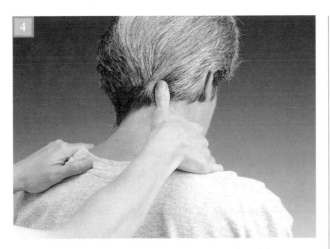

BL10, *just below the skull and to the outside of the crest of trapezius, is a neck release point that works very well on occipital headaches.*

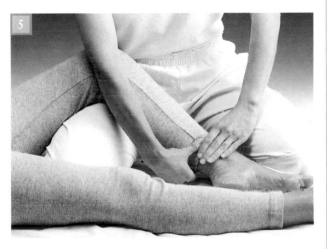

If the headaches seem to be hormonally based and occur around period time, SP6 is the most effective point. Used every day, it can regulate hormonal imbalances.

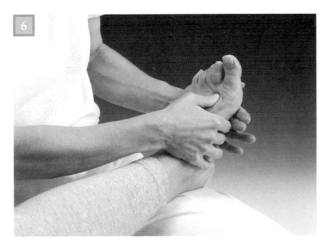

The classic tsubo to use in the case of one-sided migraines or severe headaches manifesting on the Gall Bladder meridian in the head – LIV3.

accompanied by tightness on one side of the neck. Tension in the jaw also frequently causes head pain, and is often symptomatic of the "biting your tongue" attitude that may go with bottling up emotions and feeling inner frustration. The trapezius muscle located in the upper back, shoulders, and neck is another prime area for holding tension, and produces headaches in the occipital region (at the back of the head).

Our emotions are a major cause of headaches (including migraines). These headaches are described in Traditional Chinese Medicine as "Liver-Yang rising" and usually are felt as a one-sided pain on the temple, behind one eye, or on the side of the head. Worry is another source of headache, often affecting the Stomach meridian in the front of the face.

Diet is another important factor in headaches, especially migraines. Not only does the quality and quantity of food have to be considered, but also the intake of liquids. Dehydration, for example, can easily be a trigger for a severe headache, and harms the kidneys and the lungs. Indeed, the first line of action to take if you feel a headache coming on is to drink a couple of glasses of pure spring water. Many people take most of their regular liquids in the form of tea or coffee, which is bad news if you are susceptible to headaches.

Eating irregularly is another cause. Often fuzzy, front-of-head headaches are caused by low blood-glucose levels, which can occur if you go for too long without eating. This often if you're working hard and skip meals; try to eat nourishing snacks little and often, even if you don't stop for a full meal.

Various trigger foods should be avoided by many migraine sufferers. It is worth noting that many of the known triggers contain the yeastlike fungus Candida Albicans. Many cases of chronic migraines respond well to the anticandida diet, which is basically no sugar, no yeast, and no alcohol.

Finally, medication, particularly the birth control pill and Hormone Replacement Therapy, can contribute to headaches and migraines. Long-term use of either can upset the balance between Kidney and Liver meridians.

6 Bladder Problems

Bladder problems can be uncomfortable and embarrassing. The ones most usually seen in Shiatsu practice are cystitis (in both men and women) and enlarged prostate (in men). The Bladder and Kidney meridians, and the Lower Heater of the Triple Heater, are all involved in these.

Cystitis is a bacterial infection of the bladder, its symptoms being frequent and difficult urination accompanied by an acute burning sensation. The standard orthodox treatment is with antibiotics, which is fine if bacteria are actually present in the bladder and urine. However, quite often the patient just suffers from annoyingly frequent and scanty urination. In such cases, bacteria may not be present in the bladder, and, if so, taking antibiotics may actually make the condition worse.

In all cases of cystitis, there is, in energetic terms, an invasion of the bladder by dampness (causing difficulty in urinating and cloudiness of the urine), and heat (producing the hot or burning sensations). Specific points to use for this condition are CV3 and BL28: the Bo and Yu points for the Bladder. Also use SP6, which removes heat and dispels damp from the Lower Heater, and SP9, which has a general function in draining damp and removing heat from the Lower Heater.

Enlargement of the prostate affects many men over the age of 50. Its main symptom is a frequent need to urinate, with dribbling from the penis afterward. There is often a sore back and a feeling of coldness. In energy terms, this is a chronic case of Kidney meridian deficiency, and the aim of treatment is therefore to strengthen the kidneys and open the water passageways to allow fluids (in this case urine) to flow easily and smoothly. Dampness may also be a causative factor and should be addressed during treatment. Specific tsubo to work are BL23 (the Kidney Yu point), GV4, and CV4 to strengthen the Kidneys; BL28 (the Bladder Yu point) to open the water passageways and assist the flow of urine; and SP6 and SP9 to clear up dampness from the Lower Heater.

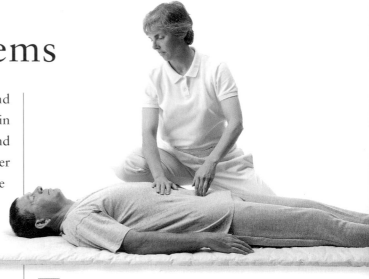

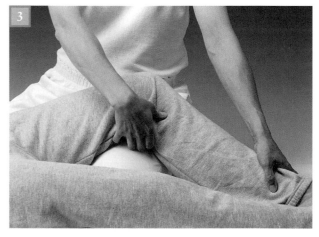

1 *CV3, the Bo point for the Bladder, is located four thumbs' width below the navel. It can be used in any sort of bladder disturbance but is particularly effective for cystitis.*

While CV3 (four thumbs' width below the navel on the midline) works principally on the Bladder, CV4 (three thumbs' width below the navel) directly affects the Kidneys.

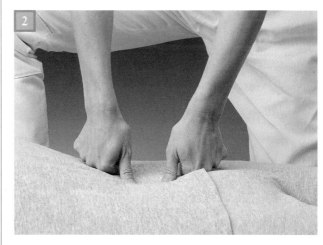

SP6 (four fingers'-width above the highest point of the inner ankle) and SP9 (just below the inside of the knee) both have the effect of removing dampness.

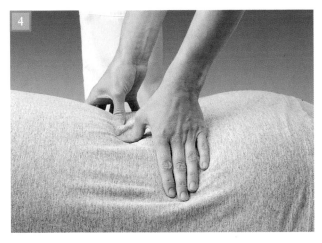

The Yu point for the kidneys, BL23, is located 1.5 cun from the midline of the spine, level with the space between the spinous processes of the second and third lumbar vertebrae. It is a strong point for tonifying the kidneys.

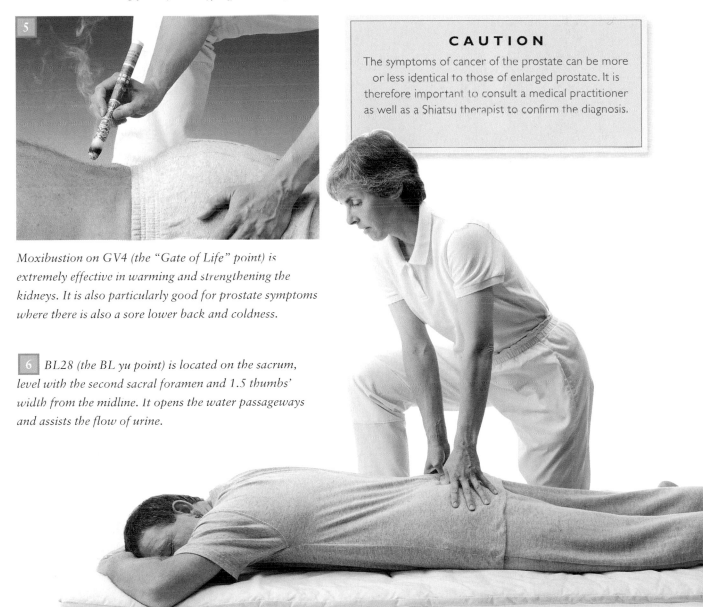

Moxibustion on GV4 (the "Gate of Life" point) is extremely effective in warming and strengthening the kidneys. It is also particularly good for prostate symptoms where there is also a sore lower back and coldness.

6 *BL28 (the BL yu point) is located on the sacrum, level with the second sacral foramen and 1.5 thumbs' width from the midline. It opens the water passageways and assists the flow of urine.*

MERIDIAN

In the Triple Heater, the Lower Heater is involved in bladder problems, since it comprises the excretory functions and the meridians LI, SI, BL, KD, and LIV. One of the functions of the Triple Heater is to promote the flow of Ki in the water passageways. The Bladder and Kidney meridians are concerned with the production and excretion of urine, and, in the case of the kidney, with storing our essential vitality and Jing. The Kidney meridian is thus often affected in bladder complaints.

CAUTION

The symptoms of cancer of the prostate can be more or less identical to those of enlarged prostate. It is therefore important to consult a medical practitioner as well as a Shiatsu therapist to confirm the diagnosis.

⁊ How to Find a Practitioner

Over the past fifteen years, complementary and alternative therapies have enjoyed a remarkable rise in popularity. Disillusionment with the drug-based treatment of orthodox medical practice, coupled with a lack of time on the part of family doctors and an increasing desire by patients to play a more active and responsible role in their own treatment have all, no doubt, played their part in turning a great many people toward much gentler systems of medicine.

It is within the scope of most natural therapies to give patients an understanding of their conditions in relation to their overall health potential, and perhaps it is this quest for self-understanding and the need for some sympathetic person with a different outlook and sufficient time to talk over health concerns that leads so many people to try these therapies. However, once you are away from the established norms of orthodox medicine, there is the very real question of standards and qualifications. How can you find a reputable practitioner? Is there a national regulatory organization? Is it best to approach a training school for their list of therapists? Do all schools train to the same standard? For the unfortunate patient who only wants someone to ease his back pain, it can seem like a wilderness.

Most countries in the West now have professional societies that encompass all practitioners, teachers, and students of Shiatsu. They unite everyone with an active interest in Shiatsu and work to promote all aspects of the therapy, from providing public information to setting standards of professional practice within the particular territory in which each society or organization operates.

ABOVE *A good teacher of Shiatsu will have a sympathetic personality and proper accreditation.*

The Shiatsu Society in Great Britain was born out of an initiative in 1981, when a small group of teachers and students of Shiatsu met to discuss ways of forging links between the few pioneers involved in the therapy in Britain at that time. Originally conceived as a communications network, it soon took on the role of professional association and information point for the public, and published a register of practitioners. The setting of standards for professional training and practice was seen as the responsibility of the existing senior teachers and practitioners. This resulted in discussions to set up a system to unify standards that would respect each individual practitioner's unique way of working, and would take into account the varying styles and philosophical approaches taught by different training establishments.

The Shiatsu Society, therefore, acts as an umbrella organization for Shiatsu in Britain. In Europe, several countries have formed similar organizations and these now communicate and collaborate on matters of mutual interest through the European Shiatsu Federation. For example, they have lobbied to have Shiatsu specifically named as a non-conventional medical discipline in the Lannoye Report on the status of non-conventional medicine in the European Union. Australia has its own professional body, the Shiatsu Therapy Association of Australia, while in the United States, therapists come together with practitioners of other Eastern-based healing methods under the American Bodywork Therapy Association. The development of the A.O.B.T.A. more or less mirrors that of the Shiatsu Society in Britain,

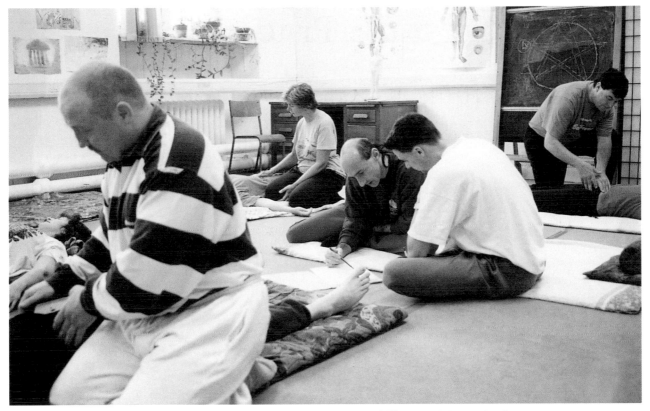

ABOVE *A Shiatsu training session in progress. The instructor is demonstrating one-handed hara diagnosis (see p. 136).*

although the methods for accrediting training establishments are somewhat different. Addresses for all these organizations, as well as those in Japan, are given on page 190.

One of the guiding principles behind all these societies has always been to encourage communication between practitioners and teachers of different styles and approaches to Shiatsu, in an effort to avoid the disagreements that have dogged other therapies from time to time.

All the major Shiatsu schools are run by Registered Teacher members of the Shiatsu Society, and graduates from the schools are eligible to sit the Society's practitioner assessment, which governs entry to the Register of Practitioners. This Register is a unified listing of practitioners from different training establishments who have completed a minimum of three years' training, have passed their school's qualifying examinations, and have satisfied the Society's Assessment Panel of their professional competence in both practical and theoretical work. Registered Practitioners may use the letters M.R.S.S. (Member of the Register of the Shiatsu Society).

ACCREDITATION

At the present time, all the national associations have individual, though broadly similar, standard requirements, covering the theory and practice of Shiatsu, and the length and intensity of study that govern entry to the relevant national Therapists Register; obviously the fine detail of accreditation varies from country to country. Accreditation by independent national agencies is an issue being addressed by most of the Shiatsu organizations worldwide, and is seen by many professional Shiatsu therapists as the way forward in having Shiatsu more widely accepted as a bona fide profession.

If you are seriously considering training to become a Shiatsu practitioner, you are strongly advised only to work with a teacher or within a school or college that has full accreditation from the appropriate Shiatsu association for the country in which you live. Poor instruction may lead to inadequate practice, and this will not only be unsatisfactory for your clients but could even prove potentially dangerous.

⑧ Training in Shiatsu

Classes in Shiatsu are fairly widely available in Britain and the U.S., either as leisure interest evening classes at beginner level, or as professional training for those who wish to become practicing therapists. Most classes are held on evenings or weekends, although one or two of the large colleges run day-time professional courses. Although not yet as widespread as instructors in, for example, yoga, it is usually not too difficult to find a Shiatsu teacher local to you. Details of courses can be obtained from your national Shiatsu society and in Britain they are often advertised in the Shiatsu Society's quarterly newsletter.

Training in Shiatsu is not merely a question of learning the theory and techniques. As I have emphasized throughout this book, Shiatsu is about attitude, self-understanding, and personal development. If you are serious in your intention to become a practitioner, I strongly suggest that you find a teacher or organization you feel you can trust and grow with – you may need to try several beginners' classes before you find someone you really "click" with.

Most schools do not have entrance requirements other than enthusiasm and motivation: many try to get away from the old academic ways of working that most of us had enough of at elementary school. Classes may include a large proportion of practical hands-on work, with games, creative work, and sensitivity exercises to facilitate learning with the whole body, the senses, and the feelings, as well as the mind. Of course, intellectual effort is also needed, especially at more advanced levels, where Oriental theory, diagnosis, anatomy, physiology, and pathology form part of the curriculum. Some schools set practical and written homework, and some form of assessment is usually included at the end of a course.

Later in your training you will be encouraged to study with different teachers in order to broaden your outlook, increase your repertoire of techniques, and learn to respect other approaches to Shiatsu. Many schools run courses that take students up to national Shiatsu society standard; other individual teachers may offer classes in special aspects of Shiatsu or take pupils to certain levels before referring them on to other teachers.

Each national society provides a list of Registered Teachers and recognized Shiatsu schools. Their newsletters and other publications also provide nationwide details of classes, as well as information on special seminars with teachers from abroad.

BELOW *Shiatsu training needs a positive attitude and self-understanding as well as a trustworthy instructor.*

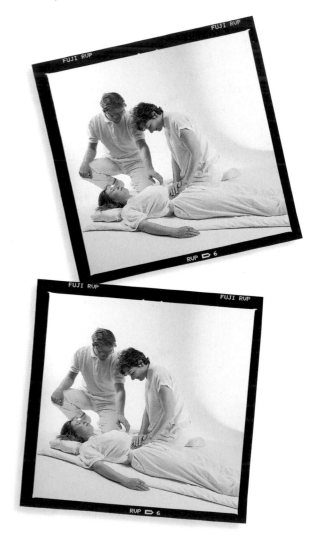

9 In Conclusion: Why Shiatsu?

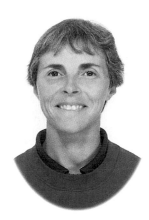

ABOVE *The author, Elaine Liechti, who is Senior Tutor at the Glasgow School of Shiatsu in Scotland, and a respected practitioner of Zen Shiatsu.*

If we look on healing as the process of becoming whole, I firmly believe that each of us has the ability to heal others, in some way, if we choose to do so. I also believe that the desire to help and heal springs from our essential humanity and sympathy for the other living beings traveling with us on this complex, confusing, sometimes joyous, and sometimes painful journey we call Life. How we choose to express our healing depends on us individually. Some of us bump into it early in life; others never manage to be tuned in sufficiently to be able to express this positive aspect of themselves.

Personally, I fell into Shiatsu almost literally, through practicing the martial art aikido. A fall on the mat and someone using tsubo to bring me around, a series of lectures on Yin Yang, and the development of ferocious migraines all led me to investigate Shiatsu for the sake of my own health. I went on a weekend course and that was it! I had found what I wanted to do in life. Here was a way that I could help others and could communicate at a deep level – having obtained a degree in languages and been involved in journalism prior to taking up Shiatsu, communication has always been important to me. At the same time, I could work on my own health and personal strength. The discipline of Shiatsu practice appealed to me, as well as the fact that it harnesses one's power through the use of hara, yet uses the power in a compassionate and nurturing way. Its movement and creativity extended both my body and mind, while my entry into the unseen world of the workings of Ki fascinated me. In short, Shiatsu as a medium for self-expression and healing was completely aligned with my own energy

quality. If I had been different, I might have found another therapy, or spiritual healing, or yoga, or conventional medicine. There is a saying in esoteric teaching: "When the pupil is ready, the master will appear." I feel that Shiatsu has been my master and teacher for many years, guiding me to self-understanding and a knowledge of my purpose in life.

I have no illusions that Shiatsu can cure all things; for me, it is more a way of holding up a mirror and letting patients take a look at themselves. Sometimes this has the effect of helping them let go of pain or a longstanding health problem, or of helping them start to care for themselves. Sometimes Shiatsu helps someone get his or her life in order sufficiently to be able to cope with problems; sometimes it can help someone to die with dignity.

The power of compassionate touch is immense. The power of healing touch, used with a knowledge of energy in a system such as Shiatsu, has the ability to enhance people's lives in a tremendously positive way. By reaching out through Shiatsu with its sympathetic, holistic approach to and improving the quality of individuals' lives, we can perhaps improve the quality of life for everyone on our earth.

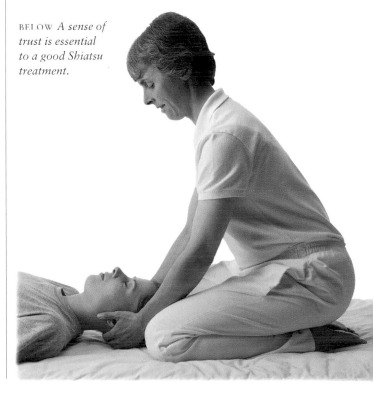

BELOW *A sense of trust is essential to a good Shiatsu treatment.*

Points: Locations and Functions

Knowing the location of tsubo is very useful for anyone wanting to extend their knowledge of Shiatsu to practitioner level, although you will need formal instruction to find out their many varied functions. Listed here are those which students of Shiatsu are expected to know for their theory exam, and they provide a useful check-list. For exact location, anatomical terms are used: if in doubt please consult a medical dictionary. Measurements are made in cun i.e. one thumb width.

LUNG MERIDIAN

LU 1: 1 cun below the hollow under the lateral end of the clavicle. LU Bo point. Regulates Lung Ki. Coughing. Asthma.

LU 9: At the lateral end of the wrist crease lateral to the radial artery. Tonifies Lung Ki. Chronic cough. Stimulates circulation.

LARGE INTESTINE MERIDIAN

LI 4: On the highest point of the web of flesh between the first and second metacarpals. Pain relief in face, head, and teeth. Sneezing, hay fever. Stimulates intestines. Promotes downward flow of Ki: promotes labor (contraindicated in pregnancy).

LI 10: 2 cun distal to the lateral end of the elbow crease. General well-being. Pain and tiredness in the arm and upper body.

LI 15: In the anterior hollow at the top of the deltoid muscle. Frozen shoulder. Pain and paralysis in the arm and shoulder.

LI 20: In the groove, level to the midpoint of nostril. Nasal congestion. Loss of sense of smell. Nose bleeds, hay fever. Facial pain.

STOMACH MERIDIAN

ST 3: Directly below the pupil, under the cheekbone, level with the nostril. Facial paralysis. Trigeminal neuralgia. Nasal obstruction.

ST 25: 2 cun lateral to the navel. LI Bo point. Abdominal pain. Diarrhea. Clears Heat from Stomach and Intestines.

ST 36: 3 cun below the hollow at the lower lateral corner of the kneecap. Tonifies Stomach and Spleen: all Stomach problems. Strengthens the body and mind.

SPLEEN MERIDIAN

SP 3: On the side of the foot, behind the joint forming the ball of the foot. Tonifies SP. Stimulates the brain. Relieves Dampness. Strengthens the spine.

SP 6: 3 cun above the tip of the medial malleolus posterior to the tibia. Strengthens and tonifies Spleen, Kidney, and Liver. Any gynecological and menstrual problems, relieves Damp. Calms the mind. Insomnia (contraindicated in pregnancy).

SP 9 On the lower border of the medial condyle of the tibia. Eliminates Dampness: diarrhea, edema in the legs. Painful and swollen knees.

SP 10: 2 cun above medial epicondyle of the femur on the bulge of inner quadriceps. Painful or irregular periods. Eczema, rashes, nettle rash.

HEART MERIDIAN

HT 7: On the medial side of the wrist crease, proximal to the pisiform bone lateral to the flexor tendon. Calms the mind. Anxiety. Insomnia. Heart problems.

HT 9: On the radial side of the tip of the little finger about 0.1 cun proximal to the nail bed. Relieves fullness in the chest. Extreme anxiety. Restores consciousness.

SMALL INTESTINE MERIDIAN

SI 3: On the ulnar side of the hand, just proximal to the head of the metacarpal. Stiff neck, headache.

SI 11: In the hollow of the center of the shoulder blade. Shoulder pain. Frozen shoulder.

SI 19: In the hollow anterior to the tragus. Deafness. Tinnitus.

BLADDER MERIDIAN

BL 2: On the notch to the medial side of the upper eye socket, or at the medial end of the eyebrow. Eye problems. Facial paralysis. Frontal headaches.

BL 10: At the base of the skull, 1.3 cun from the midline, lateral to the trapezius muscle. Occipital headache and stiff neck. Stimulates the memory. Assists eyesight. Acute lower back pain.

BL 13: (LU Yu point) 1.5 cun lateral to the lower border of the spinous process of the 3rd thoracic vertebrae. Lung problems. Bronchitis, pneumonia.

BL 14: (HG Yu point) 1.5 cun lateral to the lower border of the spinous process of the 4th thoracic vertebra. Heart conditions: coronary heart disease, angina, irregular heart beat.

BL 15: (HT Yu point) 1.5 cun lateral to the lower border of the spinous process of the 5th thoracic vertebra. Calms the mind: anxiety, insomnia. Depression. Chest pain.

BL 18: (LV Yu point) 1.5 cun lateral to the lower border of the spinous process of the 9th thoracic vertebra. Liver problems. Jaundice. Blurred vision, swollen and painful eyes.

BL 19: (GB Yu point) 1.5 cun lateral to the lower border of the spinous process of the 10th thoracic vertebra. Jaundice. Nausea, vomiting. Discomfort to the diaphragm area.

BL 20: (SP Yu point) 1.5 cun lateral to the lower border of the spinous process of the 11th thoracic vertebra. Tonifies Spleen & Stomach. Abdominal pain. Indigestion. Diarrhea. Chronic illness involving tiredness. Prolapses.

BL 21: (St Yu point) 1.5 cun lateral to the lower border of the spinous process of the 12th thoracic vertebra. Stomach problems. Indigestion, nausea. Resolves Dampness

BL 22: (TH Yu point) 1.5 cun lateral to the lower border of the spinous process of the 1st lumbar vertebra. Opens the Water passages. Regulates the transformation of fluids.

BL 23: (KD Yu point) 1.5 cun lateral to the lower border of the spinous process of the 2nd lumbar vertebra. Tonifies Kidneys and Jing: impotence, infertility, low libido. Chronic lower back pain. Deafness, tinnitus.

BL 25: (LI Yu point) 1.5 cun lateral to the lower side of the spinous process of the 4th lumbar vertebra. Constipation, diarrhea. Chronic or acute back pain.

BL 27: (SI Yu point) 1.5 cun lateral to the midline, level with the 1st sacral foramen. Small Intestine problems. Abdominal pain. Lumbar and sacral pain.

BL 28: (BL Yu point) 1.5 cun lateral to the midline, level with the 2nd sacral foramen. Bladder problems. Clears Heat & Damp from the Bladder. Lower back pain and stiffness.

BL 40: At the midpoint of the crease at the back of the knee. Acute lower back pain. Burning sensation on urination.

BL 60: In the hollow between the tip of the lateral malleolus and the Achilles tendon. Chronic back pain. Stiff and painful neck and shoulders. Headache. Childbirth: pain relief during labor.

BL 67: On the lateral side of the little toe, 0.1 cun proximal to the nail bed. Headache. Eye pain. Turning breech baby (usually moxa is applied).

KIDNEY MERIDIAN

KD 1: On the sole of the foot just proximal to the ball in line with the second toe. Tonifies the body's Yin energies. Calms the mind; extreme anxiety. Brings Ki downward. Unconsciousness.

KD 3: Midway between the tip of the medial malleolus and the Achilles tendon. Tonifies the Kidneys. Tonifies Original Ki and Jing. Chronic lower back pain. Regulates the uterus; all menstrual problems. Impotence.

KD 27: In the hollow below the medial end of the clavicle, 2 cun from the mid line. Asthma, coughing, chest pain.

HEART GOVERNOR MERIDIAN

HG 6: 2 cun proximal to the wrist crease, between the tendons. Nausea. Chest problems. Calms the mind.

HG 8: In the center of the palm between the 2nd and 3rd metacarpal bones. Calms the mind. Anxiety and nervousness. Tongue ulcers.

TRIPLE HEATER MERIDIAN

TH 5: 2 cun proximal to the crease at the back of the wrist between the radius and ulna. Fever, sore throat, ear infection, dislike of cold. Arm and shoulder pain. Migraine.

GALL BLADDER MERIDIAN

GB 1: Level with the lateral corner of the eye in the hollow just within the temple area. Eye problems; red and painful eyes, conjunctivitis. Migraine.

GB 20: Below the occiput, within the hairline, between the trapezius and the sternocleidomastoid muscles. Headache (side and back of head). Stiff neck. Dizziness. Eye problems. Tinnitus and deafness.

GB 21: On top of the shoulder, midway between the shoulder joint and the spine. Neck and shoulder

stiffness. Childbirth: helps establish contractions, retention of placenta. Stimulates lactation (contraindicated in pregnancy).

GB 24: On the nipple line, between the seventh and eighth ribs. GB Bo point. Jaundice, pain around the liver, discomfort in the upper abdomen.

GB 25: On the side of the torso, below the end of the 12th floating rib. KD Bo point. Diagnosis of KD problems. Pain in lower back and upper abdomen.

GB 30: Two thirds of the distance between the tip of the sacrum and the greater trochanter of the femur in the center of the buttock. Hip and leg pain. Sciatica. Movement problems and hemiplegia in the legs.

GB 34: In the hollow anterior and inferior to the head of the fibula. Encourages the free flow of Liver Ki. Nausea and vomiting. Relaxes the tendons generally; muscle cramps. Knee pain.

LIVER MERIDIAN

LIV 3: On the top of the foot proximal to the second joint of the big toe, between the first and second metatarsals. Migraine. Muscular cramps. Calms the mind, especially anger and frustration.

LIV 13: On the side of the abdomen below the end of the 11th floating rib. SP Bo point. Promotes the smooth flow of Liver Ki and eliminates stagnation:

indigestion, abdominal distension and belching. Tonifies ST and SP.

LIV 14: On the nipple line between the sixth and seventh ribs. LIV Bo point. Belching, nausea, vomiting. Pain and fullness in the upper abdomen and chest.

CONCEPTION VESSEL

CV 3: 4 cun below the navel. BL Bo point. Acute, painful urinary problems. Pain in lower abdomen and genitals.

CV 4: 3 cun below the navel. SI Bo point. Tonifies

Ki in the Lower Heater. Strengthens the mind and body. Tonifies blood; scanty or lack of periods. Strengthens the Kidneys: chronic illness, low energy. Calms the mind.

CV 5: 2 cun below the navel. TH Bo point. Stimulates the Lower Heater to keep water passages open and transform fluids. Fluid retention in the abdomen, painful urination, vaginal discharge.

CV 6: 1.5 cun below the navel. Tonifies Ki and Yang (especially with moxa): mental and physical

exhaustion, depression, lack of will power. Abdominal pain and distension, constipation. Removes Dampness: vaginal discharge, mucus, diarrhea.

CV 12: 4 cun above the navel. ST Bo point. Tonifies Stomach and Spleen; lack of appetite. Assists Stomach Ki to descend: belching, vomiting.

CV 17: In the middle of the sternum, level with the nipples. HG Bo point. Tonifies Ki in the chest. Breathlessness, chest pain and tightness. Hiatus hernia. Lactation.

GOVERNING VESSEL

GV 4: Between the spinous processes of the 2nd & 3rd lumbar vertebrae. Tonifies Yang, and Kidney Yang: lack of vitality, depression, feeling chilly, excessive urination, weak lower back and knees. All deficient sexual disorders.

GV 20: On the crown of the head on a line connecting tops of the ears. Clears the mind and lifts the spirits. Assists the ascending function of the Spleen: prolapses, hemorrhoids. Dizziness.

Bibliography

BEINFIELD & KORNGOLD. *Between Heaven and Earth.* Ballentine Books 1991

BERESFORD–COOKE, C. *Shiatsu Theory and Practice.* Churchill Livingstone 1996

BLAKEY, P. *The Muscle Book.* Bibliotek Books 1992

CHAITOW, L. *Soft Tissue Manipulation.* Thorsons 1980

CHENG, X. *Chinese Acupuncture & Moxibustion.* Foreign Languages Press Beijing 1987

COWMEADOW. O. *Shiatsu: A Practical Introduction.* Element Books 1998

DURCKHEIM K. VON, *Hara: The Vital Centre of Man.* Unwin Paperbacks 1962

FLAWS, B. *Prince Wen Hui's Cook.* Paradigm Publications 1983

JARMEY, C. & MOJAY, G. *Shiatsu: The Complete Guide.* Thorsons 1991

KAPTCHUK, T. *Chinese Medicine: The Web that has no Weaver.* Rider 1993

KASELLE, M. & HANNAY, P. *Touching Horses.* J.A. Allen 1995

KUSHI, M. *How to see your Health.* Japan Publications 1980

LAO TSU, *Tao Te Ching.* Trans. Man Ho Kwok, Martin Palmer, and Jay Ramsay. Element Books 1993

LEGGETT, D. *Helping Ourselves: A guide to Traditional Chinese Food Energetics.* Meridian Press 1994

LIECHTI, E. *Health Essentials: Shiatsu.* Element Books 1992

LUNDBERG, P. *The Book of Shiatsu.* Gaia Books 1992

MACIOCIA, G. *The Foundations of Chinese Medicine.* Churchill Livingstone 1989

MACIOCIA, G. *The Practice of Chinese Medicine.* Churchill Livingstone 1994

MASUNAGA, S. *Zen Imagery Exercises.* Japan Publications 1987

MASUNAGA, S. *Zen Shiatsu.* Japan Publications 1977

NAMIKOSHI, T. *The Complete Book of Shiatsu Therapy.* Japan Publications 1981

PLOSS & BARTELS. *The Women.* Heinemann (Medical) 1929

RIDOLFI, R. & FRANZEN, S. *Shiatsu for Women.* Thorsons 1996

SANDIFER, J. *Health Essentials: Acupressure.* Element Books 1997

SERIZAWA, K. *Tsubo: Vital Points for Oriental Therapy.* Japan Publications 1976

SUSUKI, S. *Zen Mind, Beginner's Mind.* Weatherhill 1970

TIRAN, D. & MACK, S. ED. *Complementary Therapies for Pregnancy & Childbirth.* Shiatsu section by E. Johnson. Bailliere Tindall 1995

TOHEI, K. *Ki in Daily Life.* Japan Publications 1978

VEITH, I. TRANS. *The Yellow Emperor's Classic of Internal Medicine.* University of California Press 1966

WILLIAMS, T. *The Complete Illustrated Guide to Chinese Medicine.* Element Books 1996

Glossary

Acupressure: a system of healing similar to Shiatsu, but concentrating more on the classical points as used in Acupuncture.

Ahshi points: any points on the body that are spontaneously painful. These may be on classical meridians, or not located on meridians at all.

Cervical: related to the neck area. There are seven cervical (or neck) vertebrae in the spine.

Chakras: major energetic centers located on the midline of the body. There are seven major chakras: Crown, Third Eye, Throat, Heart, Solar Plexus, Tanden, Base. Each has a specific area of action, e.g. the Throat relates to our ability to communicate, the Base chakra is the seat of our sexual energy.

Coccyx: the tailbone located at the base of the spine. Consists of four fused vertebrae.

Cold: one of the external or Pathogenic Factors (also translated as External Pernicious Influences) that causes disease in Traditional Chinese Medicine theory. Cold causes various symptoms involving chilliness, shivering, and pain in the joints. It adversely affects the Water Element.

Cun: the measurement by which tsubo are located. It is the distance between the two finger creases when the middle finger is bent; roughly equivalent to one thumb's width. The cun is an individual's own particular measurement, therefore it is small on a child and large on an adult.

Dampness: external pathogenic factor especially affecting the Earth Element. Yin in character, it causes heavy feelings in the head, sticky or cloudy discharges and secretions, stuffy chest or stomach. If untreated may progress to form lumps, swellings, cysts.

Deltoid: the muscle at the top of the arm which abducts the arm, i.e. lifts it away from the body.

Dragon's mouth: a technique in which the thumb and index finger are stretched wide and pressure is applied with the webbing located between them.

Dryness: external pathogenic factor affecting the Metal Element. Causes dry mouth and throat; dry, cracked skin. Constipation with dry stools.

Fire: external pathogenic factor, an extreme version of Heat. It is detrimental to the Fire Element, causing high fever, dark urine, constipation with dry stools, mouth ulcers, mental agitation, delirium.

Five Elements: (also translated as Five Phases or Five Transformations). A theory used widely in oriental medicine in which energy is described by the Elements Metal, Water, Wood, Fire, and Earth. Encompasses a theory of energy flow between Elements and a grouping of similar phenomena into correspondences.

Futon: mattress made of layers of cotton wadding. Traditionally used as a bed in Japan; rolled up during the day and used as a seat. The most comfortable and effective surface for giving Shiatsu.

Gastrocnemius: calf muscle, responsible for pointing the toe.

Gluteus maximus: large superficial muscle in the buttock that extends the thigh i.e. pushes the leg backward.

Hara: Japanese word for the abdomen, acknowledged as the centre of physical and spiritual strength; much used in Shiatsu to promote balance, sensitivity of touch, and healing power.

Heat: external pathogenic factor affecting the Fire Element adversely. It causes high temperature, sweating and thirst, headache, dry mouth, and dark urine.

Iliopsoas: a common name for the two muscles psoas major and iliacus which run from the inside surfaces of the transverse processes of the 12th thoracic to 5th lumbar vertebrae and the inside of the large hip bone and sacrum respectively, to insert on the inside of the top of the femur. Action: flexes the thigh, i.e. brings the thigh toward the body.

Jing: the vital energy stored in the kidneys which regulates our pace of growth, maturity, and ageing; also regulates our ability to reproduce.

Ki: Japanese word for energy, encompassing all phenomena in the universe but used specifically in oriental medicine to describe the energy in the body.

Kyo-jitsu: the theory used in Zen Shiatsu to describe the way in which two meridians can be in a dynamic relationship where the empty or unresponsive (kyo) meridian is causing a full or over-reactive (jitsu) meridian to manifest itself elsewhere.

Lumbar: relating to the five vertebrae of the spine which are not attached to ribs. Located around the waist area.

Macrobiotics: an oriental philosophy based upon Yin Yang as interpreted by George Ohsawa and Michio Kushi. Uses a specific form of dietary practice to balance the body, by designating foods into Yin or Yang categories.

Meridian: a pathway of energy in the body where Ki flows more strongly. Each meridian is related to one of the internal organs and is therefore called after it.

Moxa: a treatment to warm the body by burning the herb Artemesia Vulgaris (mugwort) on or over specific points. Moxibustion is usually applied by holding a cigar-like stick of moxa over a point.

Occiput: The back of the head or skull.

Piriformis: a deep buttock muscle whose action is to turn the thigh outward. This muscle is particularly prone to tension.

Sacrum: a fusion of five vertebrae at the base of the spine, the sacrum forms part of the pelvic girdle along with the hip bones.

Sacro-iliac: the joint positioned between the sacrum and the ilium (part of the hip bone).

Sternocleidomastoid (SCM): pair of large muscles running from the skull just behind the ear to the top of the sternum (breastbone) and clavicle (collarbone). Turns the head from side to side if used singly; when both used together draws the head forward.

Shen: the Spirit (also translated as Mind) referring to all the psychological and emotional elements to our individuality.

Tanden: a point three fingers' width below the navel, at the centre of Hara.

TCM – Traditional Chinese Medicine: a specific branch of oriental theory particularly used by acupuncturists.

Thoracic: relates to the chest area, particularly the 12 vertebrae that are attached to the ribs.

Third Eye: the chakra located between the eyebrows, relates to our psychic energies and abilities.

Tibia: the large shin bone in the lower leg.

Trapezius: a kite-shaped muscle covering the upper back, shoulders, and extending into the back of the skull. Has a wide range of actions including lifting and rotating the shoulderblades, flexing the neck to the side, and maintaining the spine in extension.

Trigger points: points which, when they are pressed, reflex pain to other sites in the body.

Tsubo: Japanese word for the classical points, usually to be found on meridians, although there are also some non-meridian extraordinary points.

Wind: external pathogenic factor which affects particularly the Wood Element, but may combine with other pathogenic factors to injure any of the Elements or organs. Characterized by sudden onset and symptoms which blow about the body, changing rapidly. Causes pain and stiffness in the upper body, tickly throat, runny nose, sneezing, slight fever, dislike of cold or wind.

Yin Yang: the dynamic underpinning all forms of oriental medicine, in which complementary and opposing forces interact in a never-ending flow: for example hot and cold, day and night, male and female.

Zen: a form of Buddhism which acknowledges that Enlightenment can occur at any time, encouraging spontaneity and living in the present; "being here right now."

Useful Addresses

Great Britain

The Shiatsu Society
Interchange Studios
Dalby Street
London, NW5 3NQ
Tel. 0171-813-7772

Japan

Japanese Shiatsu College
2-15-6 Koishikawa
Bunkyoku
Tokyo
Japan

Iokai Centre
1-8-9 Higashiuena
Daito-Ku
Tokyo
Japan

Eire

Shiatsu Society of Ireland
Greenville Lodge
Esker Road
Lucan
Co. Dublin

Australia

The Shiatsu Therapy Association
of Australia
332 Carlisle Street
Balclava
3183 Victoria
Australia
or
PO BOX 598
Belgrave
3160 Victoria
Australia

USA

American Oriental Bodywork
Therapy Association
50 Maple Place
Manhasset, New York 11030
USA

Europe

The European Shiatsu Federation
Piazza S.Agostino 24
20123
Milano
Italy

Index